ADVANCE PRAISE FOR THE PALEO PRIMER

*The Ultimate Health and Fitness Recipe Book! If you're serious about building a new you—a person brimming with strength, health, and vitality, with a lean, powerful, and athletic body—*The Paleo Primer *will deliver the answers! Written with wit and good humor, it takes you on a step-by-step journey to lifelong strength and health, teaching you what to eat, how to source it, and how to prepare it.*

–Brooks Kubik
Author of *Dinosaur Training: Lost Secrets of Strength and Development*
BrooksKubik.com

Science made simple. Great contribution to a healthy lifestyle and proves healthy food can be delicious!

–Laura C., United Kingdom

A must buy! Really simple and clear instructions on how to make some great, tasty, healthy meals and snacks.

–Michael Lindsay, United Kingdom

Intelligent and witty prose. This book says everything about food and health that I truly believe in, but sometimes stumble to find words to explain in easy terms myself. Only after 70 pages of this fascinating and easy-to-read nutritional background—littered with brilliantly funny illustrations and charming coffee cup stains—do we come to the 100-plus delicious recipes. Fantastically, there is not a single recipe without an accompanying mouth-watering picture.

–Ceri Jones, United Kingdom

Nothing like anything else. So far every recipe I have used has tasted awesome. I've used it for friends and family; it makes good food tasty! Simple as that. Well worth it just for the information on healthy eating at the beginning of the book.

–Mick H., United Kingdom

THE PALEO PRIMER

A JUMP-START GUIDE TO LOSING BODY FAT AND LIVING PRIMALLY!

KERIS MARSDEN AND MATT WHITMORE

THE PALEO PRIMER: A JUMP-START GUIDE TO LOSING BODY FAT AND LIVING PRIMALLY!

The Paleo Primer was adapted from the book Fitter Food, written and published in the United Kingdom by Keris Marsden and Matt Whitmore, Fitter Food, Inc., in 2013.

Library of Congress Control Number: 2013908805

Library of Congress Cataloging-in-Publication Data is on file with the publisher

Marsden, Keris 1980- ; and Whitmore, Matt 1985-

The Paleo Primer/Keris Marsden and Matt Whitmore

ISBN: 978-1-939563-04-0

1. Cooking 2. Health 3. Diet 4. Low carb

US Editor: Jessica Taylor Tudzin
US Copy Editor: Nancy Wong Bryan
Index: Gail Kearns
Book Design: Katherine Keeble (UK), Caroline De Vita (US)
US Cover Design: Janée Meadows
Illustrations: Mark Goodhead
Photography by Keris Marsden and Matt Whitmore
Additional photography by Jennifer Meier, Librakv/Shutterstock.com, AI1962/Shutterstock.com,
   Adisa/Shutterstock.com, and Anna Hoychuk/Shutterstock.com

Published in the United States by Primal Blueprint Publishing
23805 Stuart Ranch Road, Suite 145, Malibu, CA 90265

Visit our website at www.primalblueprintpublishing.com. For information on quantity discounts, please call 888-774-6259 or email info@PrimalBlueprintPublishing.com

BREAKFAST

LIGHT BITES

OUR TOP BURGER BITES

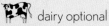 includes dairy   dairy optional

HEALTHY SNACKS

Cheats of Champions

ACKNOWLEDGMENTS

A massive thank you goes out to Mark Sisson and his staff for bringing this book to the American audience under *The Paleo Primer* name. We are beyond thrilled with your adaptation! This book was originally published in the UK under the name *Fitter Food: A Lifelong Recipe for Health and Fat Loss*. We put it together in just over four months. So many people went the extra mile and dropped everything to help us meet the rather ambitious deadline on our first version.

It could not have happened without our wonderful parents. They helped in every way possible: cooking, tasting, editing, and helping to research recipes and ingredients. To devote ourselves to that project, we reduced our working hours and moved back home to enable us to invest everything in the project. Firstly, a BIG thank you to Christine Lashmar (Matt's mom) for putting up with us invading her kitchen, and a huge congratulations to her for losing 21 pounds in the process, by eating paleo, of course! Another BIG thank you to Celine Marsden (Keris's mom), who deserves special recognition for all her hard work applying paleo principles to some of her traditional family recipes and helping to transform them into the healthy recipes featured in the book.

A big thank you to Thomas Marsden (Keris's brother) for lending us his culinary advice and expertise and assisting in the photo editing process. Words cannot even begin to describe our gratitude toward Katherine Keeble, quite simply the BEST book designer in the world! Katherine worked around the clock to make the British version of this book ready for press. She advised on everything from publication, printing, e-books, and portion size to oven temperatures and baking cookies.

Our fantastic illustrations are the work of Mark Goodhead, aka Mr. Sketchy. You can check out more of his work at CargoCollective.com/mrsketchy. We would also personally like to thank nutritionist Calum Gore of Unique Nutritionists for mentoring us through the science behind digestive well-being and food intolerance testing. More details can be found at mrtuk.co.uk. Furthermore, we'd like to thank the fantastic lecturers at the College of Naturopathic Medicine, with an extra special thank you to Fiona Hyams and Emma Mihill for simply being inspirational Naturopaths.

We wish to thank all our Fitter London members, a bunch of totally cool people committed to health and fitness as a lifestyle. Their spirit and enthusiasm provides us with daily inspiration and makes our job totally awesome.

We are truly blessed to be surrounded by such amazing, talented people on both sides of the pond!

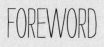

FOREWORD

In the past several years, there have been a number of outstanding books written by the leading voices in the ancestral health movement, including Robb Wolf, Gary Taubes, Loren Cordain, and dare I say myself with *The Primal Blueprint* (which took two years to research and write). Books by these and other authors convey the ancestral principles in great detail and with excellent scientific support.

While the knowledge base and the expert voices of the movement are growing impressively, cutting to the chase can be quite appealing to those of us who lead busy lives and are looking for direct, easy-to-follow guidance. Many simply want to know what, why, and how to improve dietary habits, implement exercise strategies, and comprehend general health in the ancestral model. With *The Paleo Primer*, our friends across the pond, Matt Whitmore and Keris Marsden, have done a masterful job doing just that, creating a fun, extremely creative, and informative book to help you get healthier and enjoy the process.

You can feel the passion and personality come through the pages as Keris and Matt each relate their health struggles despite striving to lead fit, athletic lives. The exploration, awakening, and health breakthroughs they achieved form the backbone of this book, and why it is certain to have a deep impact on you. Yep, even if some well-meaning loved one handed this to you in good faith and you are now holding it skeptically, you can't help but take notice, take a second look, and take stock of what you are currently doing that can get a whole lot better.

Just for fun, take a quick spin through all the pages before you settle in for a proper read. That's what I did, and in only a few moments, I could tell it was something special. I guarantee that you'll be drawn in by the clever visuals, the simple format, and the compelling points they make page after page. Often, Keris and Matt dispense healthy doses of that British wit that will leave you smiling—and remembering the salient points—long after a page is turned!

It's my great pleasure on behalf of the Primal Blueprint Publishing team to share this book with as many readers as possible. I sure hope you have as much fun as I did reading it, and as Matt and Keris did writing it!

In good health,

MARK SISSON
Malibu, CA
May 2013

THE PALEO PRIMER

> *Eighty percent of your body composition is determined by what you eat.* —**MARK SISSON,** *The Primal Blueprint*

INTRODUCTION

Welcome to *The Paleo Primer*. We want to inspire you to make some simple nutritional changes that will have a huge effect on your health, confidence, and appearance. No matter what your particular goals, focusing on your health will increase your chances of success. So whether you're looking to lose weight, build lean muscle mass or a six-pack, obtain a quicker 10k time, or turn back the hands of time (good nutrition can be incredibly anti-aging!), the principles outlined in this book will help get you there. We've kept the information simple, the science straightforward, and the recipes exciting, so that by the time you have finished reading this book, you'll be itching to get started in the kitchen.

When it comes to food, we understand that convenience sometimes take precedence over eating healthily. But the two don't have to be mutually exclusive. This book is packed with more than a hundred incredibly tasty and healthful meals, snacks, and cakes (yes, cakes!) that you can put together in minutes!

We've seen first hand how people successfully adopt a healthier lifestyle when they understand the basics of nutrition. For this reason, the first half of this book is devoted to expert advice on the subject. You'll then be ready to get cracking in the kitchen, and so the second half of this book is loaded with recipes to get you started, along with our recommendations on how to learn more and where and how to source ingredients!

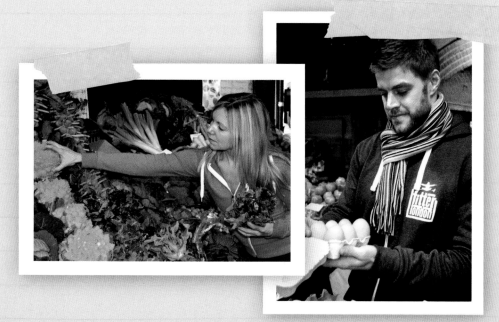

ABOUT US

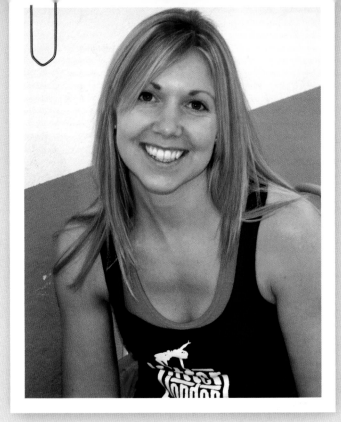

KERIS MARSDEN

After completing a diploma in public health nutrition, I entered the fitness industry as a personal trainer. During a trip to Sweden, I attended a nutrition course run by strength coach Charles Poliquin, who opened my eyes to the value of alternative and functional medicine and how they play a key role in nutritional therapy. I went on to study naturopathic nutrition at the London College of Naturopathic Medicine. My approach to nutrition was further informed by research on ancestral health and evolution. I urge you to check out the books and websites recommended in the back of this book. Each one of these resources has played a profound role in my professional development.

Before studying nutrition as a discipline, I, like most women, was completely guided by the expert marketing of the food and diet industry. I tried every diet out there, wasting hours counting calories and avoiding fat. In fact, I'd probably have eaten paper if you stamped "fat free" on it!

Back in those days, I faced a constant battle maintaining my weight. Exercise seemed like the obvious place to start my exploration into health and fitness. I was motivated to learn more in my early twenties, however, when I suffered a terrible bout of acne and was diagnosed with a common hormonal disorder called polycystic ovarian syndrome (PCOS). Although the antibiotics and birth control pills I was treated with helped clear my acne, I was concerned that they only treated the symptoms of my PCOS without addressing the underlying cause. Also, to add insult to injury, the antibiotics left me with dreadful digestive issues, and it was not very long before I was diagnosed with irritable bowel syndrome (IBS).

I soon realized in the course of my naturopathic studies how much nutrition influences our hormones. I discovered that many of the foods I had considered nutritious were actually further aggravating my health issues. Armed with new knowledge, I swapped my cereal and soy milk for whole, natural, unprocessed foods, and the transformation was incredible: my digestion improved, my energy levels balanced, and slowly but surely my skin cleared. And my PCOS disappeared!

Maintaining a healthy weight is now effortless, and I often receive compliments about my complexion. With my transformation, my biggest realization was personally experiencing how diet plays a much larger role on body composition than exercise. I still love to train, but now I only need a couple of sessions in the gym each week—leaving me with lots more time to geek away with my nutrition books.

MATT WHITMORE

I'm a personal trainer, strength coach, and a food lover with a particular fondness for bacon and ice cream. I started training at the age of ten, thanks to my grandad, a mountain of a man who always stressed the importance of being strong and eating well. He gave me two cans of baked beans and told me to curl them a hundred times. The rest was history as my passion for training only grew.

I also love sports and played high-level rugby from a young age. Unfortunately, I had to give up rugby due to a series of injuries. Now I channel my passion for sports and self-improvement into Fitter London, a business Keris and I share that aims to help others become better in mind and body through training and nutrition.

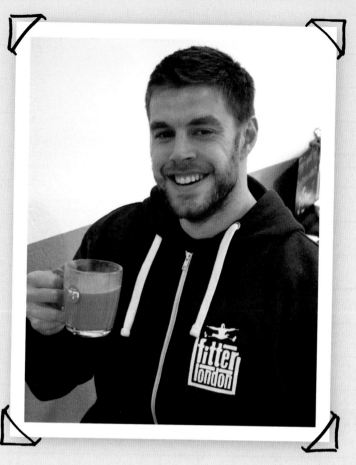

I've always been lean, and in my earlier days, didn't pay a huge amount of attention to what I put into my body. I thought nothing of wolfing down a pizza and downing ten pints of beer after a match. I now realize how incredibly naïve I was about my diet and its essential role in supporting my level of physical activity. That was after my body gave me some serious warning signs that something was amiss. I broke out in rashes, felt bloated and lethargic all the time, and my training suffered. My joints began to feel painful, and I was plagued with injury after injury. Eventually I was diagnosed with candida, a systemic yeast infection that was likely caused by my poor diet and high stress levels. It isn't life threatening, but believe me you don't want it.

This was a big turning point for me, since candida is largely treated by diet. So, all sugar and processed foods were out, and there was a big emphasis placed on increasing herbs, spices, and vegetables that have an anti-candida effect.

Finding new recipes and meal ideas had suddenly become a huge priority. If I didn't enjoy my meals, I knew I would never stick to the plan. Anyone who knows me knows that **I love food and I eat a lot!** I'm glad I didn't have to sacrifice that. This sounds incredibly cheesy, but changing my diet literally changed my life. The bloating disappeared, my energy levels soared, and my training went to a whole new level. I felt amazing! And once you experience that, you don't ever want to go back. I gained all this through eating amazing, tasty food that's nothing but good for you.

I am a changed man ... but still a bacon lover, of course.

CHAPTER 1

WHAT IS THE PALEO DIET?

❞ I saw results—lasting ones—and I've discovered so many tasty new foods, sweet potato being the best. I've never had a six-pack before. Finally I have one. But best of all, I know how to keep it. ***FRANCISSCO CUSSIANO*** (Client) **❞**

The paleo diet is about eating real food. By real food, we mean food in its natural state that has not undergone any processing or manufacturing. Essentially, this is meat, poultry, fish, eggs, natural fats, vegetables, fruit, nuts, seeds, herbs, and spices. Quite simply we want you to eat like a caveman ... with a modern twist.

We're asking you to "eat like a caveman" because the Paleolithic Era was a time when mankind thrived. Our earliest ancestors were physically strong and virtually disease free, thanks in no small part to the foods they ate. You may hear different names for this nutritional approach—Primal, the ancestral human diet, evolutionary eating, the caveman diet. Lately, we been hearing it called Paleo 2.0. We simply like to call it "fitter foods."

Every recipe in this book is designed to fuel a healthy Primal/paleo lifestyle and is packed with nutrients without compromising on taste. To this approach, we've also added some dairy products such as quality cheese, butter, and heavy cream (whipping cream or half and half). Even though these foods didn't appear until the Neolithic Era, they contain incredibly healthy fats and other nutrients, so we felt they deserve a place on the table for those who don't suffer from lactose intolerance or casein sensitivities.

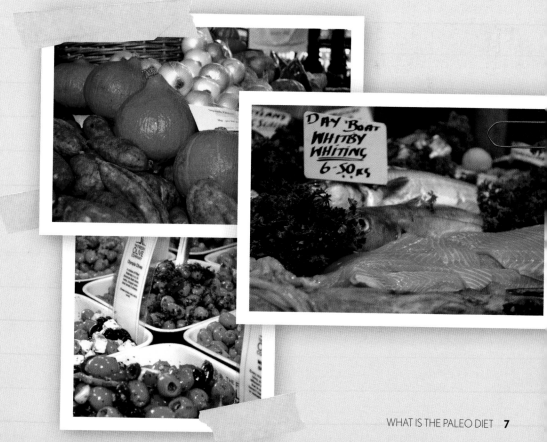

WE KNOW WHAT YOU'RE THINKING...

We've evolved!

While this may be true, our need to eat as our Paleolithic ancestors did is actually even greater than ever! Busy lifestyles, working long hours, and juggling family and friends can often leave us stressed, time poor, and reaching for convenience foods. Over time, this lethal combination has not only expanded our waistlines, but has also resulted in a rapid decline of our overall health.

To combat the detrimental effects of modern-day living, we need to fill our plates with natural foods—abundant in healthy fats, antioxidants, vitamins, and minerals—that have fueled the human race for over two million years. There is no diet richer in these than the human diet that existed back in the BC era—and by BC, we mean "Before Crap!"

Didn't cavemen die before the age of 35?

The average mortality rate in the Paleolithic Era is generally skewed because, without modern medicine, many died at birth or shortly thereafter. Furthermore, even a minor trauma, such as a broken bone, often meant sure death. Naturally, with the advent of modern medicine, human life expectancy has increased dramatically in the last century. But though we may be living longer, we are not thriving in our old age.

Meat, eggs, butter... all that fat! What about my cholesterol levels?

Yes, our recipes include saturated fat, red meat, eggs, and butter. Concerned? We aren't surprised, but there's absolutely no need to be. Unfortunately, many health claims that we read and hear about are often driven more by political or economic gain than by a sincere interest in public health. Many claims are not even substantiated with reliable science. Correlation does not mean causation, but that is exactly the sort of conclusion that has been drawn with many widely cited studies. For years we have believed that consuming foods high in saturated fat and cholesterol would clog our arteries and increase our risk of heart disease. However, newer studies have completely discredited this heart-health hypothesis, simply because the threat never existed. Three large cohort studies (the Framingham Study,[1] the Honolulu Heart Program Study,[2] and the Japanese Lipid Intervention Trial[3]) have all concluded that, in fact, having low cholesterol actually increases your risk of cardiovascular disease.[4] Furthermore, there is no statistically significant correlation between diseases like heart disease and saturated fat.[5]

---

[1] The Framingham Study, FraminghamHeartStudy.org.
[2] I. Schatz, K. Masaki, K. Yano, R. Chen, B. Rodriguez, C. Curb ,"Cholesterol and all-cause mortality in elderly people from the Honolulu Heart Program: a cohort study," *The Lancet*, vol. 358 (2001), 351-355.
[3] A. Okyama, H. Ueshim, M. Marmot, M. Yamakara, M. Nakamura, Y. Kitay, Y. Masanobu, "Changes in Total Serum Cholesterol and Other Risk Factors for Cardiovascular Disease in Japan, 1980-1989," *International Journal of Epidemiology*, vol. 22 (2003), 1038-1047.
[4] P. Siri-Tarino, Q. Sun, F. Hu, R. Krauss, "Meta-analysis of prospective cohort studies evaluating the association of saturated fat with cardiovascular disease," *American Journal of Clinical Nutrition*, vol. 91 (2010) 535-46.
[5] Neurobiologist Stephan Guyenet provides an excellent review at WholeHealthSource.blogspot.co.uk/2011/01/does-dietary-saturated-fat-increase.html

Clever marketing campaigns by the food industry have added further confusion by convincing us that all fat is the enemy, and we should be living on low-fat cereals, crackers, and whole-grain bread. Pharmaceutical companies have also had a powerful influence, as they supply the drugs to "fix" us when these foods make us sick. And sometimes they try to fix us when we're not sick.

Cholesterol, for example, is and always has been a vital nutrient to the human body. As with saturated fat, cholesterol does not cause heart disease.[6] This is exciting news as it means bacon and eggs for breakfast is a healthier choice than low-fat muesli and whole-grain toast. This topic really is a book within itself. If you are keen to know more, we suggest reading Dr. Roger Murphee's book *Heart Disease: What Your Doctor Won't Tell You*, so that you can have an educated response when your physician tells you your cholesterol is too high. New, cutting-edge studies are now establishing that other factors in our diet like sugar[7] and excessive omega-6 fats[8] (detailed in Chapter 4) actually play a much greater role in the progression of heart disease.

Before moving on, we would like to emphasize one last point: the quality of your food is paramount. In Chapter 8, we will detail the best of the best ingredients for optimal health.

Medicine is not healthcare. Food is health care. Medicine is sick care. *UNKNOWN*

WHY EAT PALEO FOOD?

Put simply, it will enhance your quality of life. You will look great, feel amazing, live longer, and have ...

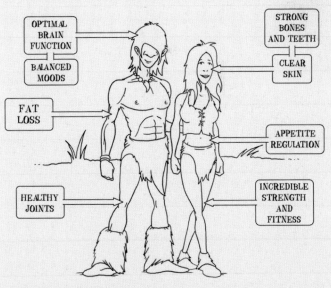

OPTIMAL BRAIN FUNCTION

BALANCED MOODS

FAT LOSS

HEALTHY JOINTS

STRONG BONES AND TEETH

CLEAR SKIN

APPETITE REGULATION

INCREDIBLE STRENGTH AND FITNESS

[6] The Framingham Study showed that those with cholesterol levels below 140 were most likely to die from cardiovascular disease, while those with levels at 240 were less likely.
[7] A. Barclay, P. Petocz, J. McMillan-Price, V. Flood, T. Prvan, P. Mitchell, and C. Brand-Miller "Glycemic index, glycemic load, and chronic disease risk–a meta analysis of observational studies." *American Journal of Clinical Nutrition*, vol. 87 (2008), 627-37.
[8] J. Hibbeln, L. Nieminen, T. Blasbalg, J. Riggs, W. Lands, "Healthy intakes of n–3 and n–6 fatty acids: estimations considering worldwide diversity." *American Journal of Clinical Nutrition*, vol. 83 (2006), 1483-1493S.

CHAPTER 2

SIGNS YOUR DIET IS NOT WORKING

So many of us are obsessed with losing weight, but the truth is we should be focusing more on our health in general. Our bodies are pretty darn good at sending us warning signals when things aren't running as they should be. But all too often we ignore these signals or, even worse, consider them to be normal. It's time to start listening to what our bodies have to say. Let's take a look at a few common telltale signs.

1. YOU'RE STORING BODY FAT!

Excuse us for stating the obvious, but a lot of folks ignore the fact that they need to lose a few pounds! It's becoming a global problem, especially since most nations have become industrialized. The World Health Organization (WHO) predicts that by 2015, there will be 2.3 billion overweight adults, and more than 700 million of them will be obese.[9] In fact, we are already seeing an increase in a variety of weight-related health problems in areas around the world that have never before experienced such a thing.

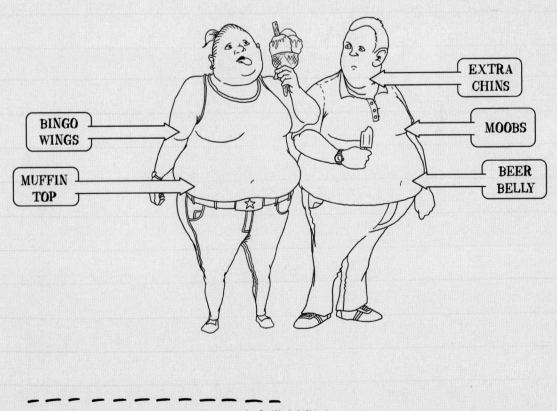

[9] World Health Organization, www.who.int/chp/chronic_disease_report/part2_ch1/en/index16.html

THE SCIENCE BIT - BODY COMPOSITION

We are genetically designed to move and stay active throughout the day. However, most people nowadays have sedentary jobs that involve being stuck at a desk and working ridiculously long hours. On top of this, we have cars, escalators, and remote controls that further encourage us to move less. Meanwhile, our diets are more energy-dense than ever, thanks to processed, packaged, and prepared foods. We're talking about boxed cereals, bagged chips, sweet snacks in wrappers, luncheon meats, and frozen microwave meals. These fake foods are cheap and more convenient than cooking at home with fresh produce, but there is certainly a price to pay. Most are packed with sugar, poor-quality fats, and preservatives and chemicals that we as humans were never designed to eat, and our guts never built to process. They disrupt our hormones and destroy our metabolism. Metabolism is the rate at which your body burns off and utilizes calories, so anything that impairs that process will cause chronic weight gain.

2. YOU'RE A SERIAL SNOOZER

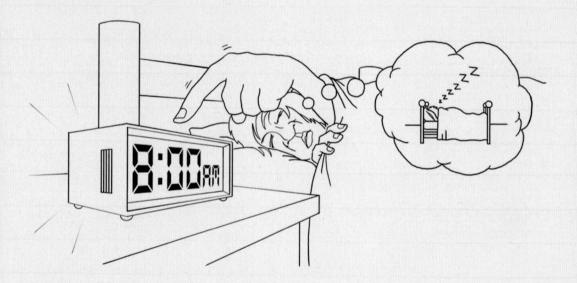

The way you feel in the morning is a good indication of your overall health. Ideally, our bodies should awaken us naturally after eight hours of restful sleep. We shouldn't even need alarm clocks—impossible to imagine, eh? Our energy levels are naturally at their highest first thing in the day, which means we should be able to kick-start our daily routines full of vitality.

Yet waking abruptly from slumber by some painful sounding alarm clock is the reality for most. We press the snooze button at least three times just to get over the shock, then spend the next ten minutes trying to figure out which part of our daily personal hygiene routines can be sacrificed to maximize pillow hugging time. After finally admitting defeat and staggering out of bed, the only thing on our minds is securing a continuous drip feed of caffeine to get us through the day until we can be reunited with our beloved beds.

THE SCIENCE BIT – HORMONE HEALTH

Early morning fatigue is a sign that your hormones are not functioning optimally, in particular those responsible for governing blood sugar levels (insulin) and "get up and go" (cortisol). These hormones play a huge role in determining your cycles of energy throughout the day and are affected by several factors, including your stress levels, sleep quality, physical activity, and yes, even what you eat and drink. The beauty of hormones is that they are like an orchestra, working together to produce the symphony that is your day. Once an instrument (or hormone) gets out of sync, however, the overall performance languishes, and other hormones soon begin to falter, including those governing reproduction, sleep, and digestion. This leads to common issues such as premenstrual syndrome (PMS), polycystic ovarian syndrome (PCOS), irritable bowel syndrome (IBS), and—horrifyingly—a lack of libido.

3. YOU FART... A LOT!

Deny it as much as you like, but we all do it. As funny as a good fart is, excessive wind is a sure sign that some of the foods you are eating are aggravating your digestive system. Besides, there's only so many times you can blame the dog.

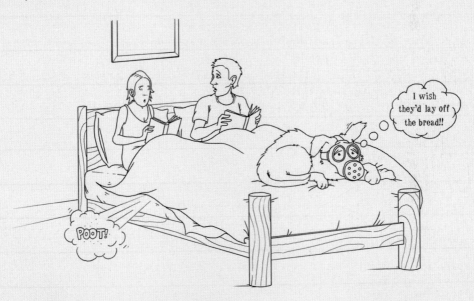

THE SCIENCE BIT – DIGESTIVE HEALTH

In her book *Detoxify or Die*, Sherry A. Rogers, a medical doctor specializing in environmental medicine, puts it this way: The road to health is paved with good intestines. Indeed, good digestive health is so much more important than most people realize!

Sadly, IBS is now a very common condition. Symptoms range from stomach cramps, flatulence, and bloating to diarrhea and constipation. Most of us experience these on a daily basis and simply consider them to be normal. In fact, this is your body's way of telling you it is none too pleased with what you're putting inside it. Many of the modern-day convenience foods we eat are highly processed and cause digestive discomfort. This is a signal you should not overlook, because your entire metabolism starts in your gut. Therefore, any issues with digestion compromise your metabolic efficiency. Furthermore, because you cannot absorb nutrients from your food effectively, poor digestive heath will often lead to some form of malnourishment and vitamin or mineral deficiency.

Poor digestion also affects your immune system. Did you know 85 percent of your immune system is situated in the gut? Our guts are designed to protect us and act as a barrier between the outside world and the body. Yet some of the foods we eat are so aggravating they can actually create microscopic gaps along the gut wall that allow food particles, bacteria, toxins, and other substances to pass into the body. The bombardment of these strange substances confuses the immune system and sends it into overdrive, leading to all sorts of health complications.

This condition is known as leaky gut syndrome, and it isn't something you should ignore. Your digestive health is your life force. Imagine a car with a leaking gas tank; no matter how much you fill up the tank, it will still eventually run out of fuel and come to a grinding halt. This is effectively what happens to the body, and symptoms soon go beyond digestive irritation to include much more serious conditions, including chronic fatigue, fever, arthritis, eczema, asthma, and migraines.

4. SKIN ISSUES

Have you ever noticed how much your skin suffers after a heavy weekend of eating and drinking? If you look in the mirror and see blemishes, wrinkles, dry skin, oily skin, a dull complexion, or dark circles under your eyes, then this could be your body's cry for help. Inflammatory skin conditions like acne, eczema, psoriasis, and dermatitis are even more serious. Often we try to treat these topically with creams and lotions, but the root cause is beyond skin deep. In fact, a strong link exists between leaky gut syndrome and skin problems.

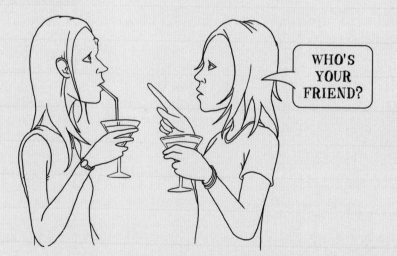

THE SCIENCE BIT - DETOXIFICATION AND INFLAMMATION
Think of your skin as a true reflection of your health. Your skin is your body's largest detoxification organ, so if it's erupting, that is a sign of toxic overload. And let's face it: we're exposed to toxins on a daily basis. Just think of the pollution, medications, and chemicals that have all made their way into our food and water supply! If your gut is unable to protect you from these toxins, the result often manifests in your skin.

THE SOLUTION: HEAL FROM THE INSIDE OUT

The message here is that the only way to achieve and, more importantly, sustain a healthy body is to start your transformation from the inside. You can buy pills and potions to treat the signs of a poor diet, but ultimately you'll need to address the root cause of the problem. Let your healthy diet act as your medicine, and you will begin to see the following dramatic changes.

BALANCED BLOOD SUGAR LEVELS

The single most important aim of your nutrition should be to balance your blood sugar levels! A diet rich in refined and processed foods works against this goal by suddenly spiking your blood sugar levels. Replace them with whole, natural foods that provide a slow, steady release of nutrients, and you'll help regulate hormones and fat storage.

DIGESTIVE SUPPORT

Now that we've explained the importance of digestive health, you can understand why it is imperative to reduce or remove gut-irritating foods. The usual suspects are highly refined grains, especially those containing gluten.

REDUCED INFLAMMATION

Most degenerative diseases—including heart disease, cancer, and diabetes—are increasing at an alarming rate around the globe. The culprit behind these diseases is inflammation within the body, something that can be hugely moderated with proper nutrition.

IMPROVED DETOXIFICATION

Our livers are quite frankly overwhelmed with toxins from our environment. Nutrition is meant to boost liver function, not burden it further with food toxins such as refined sugars, refined carbohydrates, chemical preservatives, additives, synthetic hormones, or antibiotics found in intensively farmed meat or fish. Conversely, whole, natural, and nutrient-dense foods—such as vegetables, fruits, herbs, and spices—all support liver detoxification.

So, how can nutrition achieve all that? It's easier than you think. Read on ...

CHAPTER 3

CHANGE YOUR MIND, CHANGE YOUR HEALTH

" The kick-start for me was to have a lean, toned body for my holiday in Ibiza, but once I got started I couldn't stop! I loved how I looked and felt, and rather than return to my old ways, this became a lifestyle not a diet for me. *ELIZABETH SHEPHERD* (Client) **"**

Before we delve into the basics of nutrition, it's important to understand our relationship with food. Eating well can often prove to be a psychological battle. Many of us eat to relieve stress, to feel comfort, and to deal with boredom. Tempting food is so readily available to us that we constantly have to fight our caveman instincts to eat everything in sight! So let's start by getting your mind in the right place. Your mind is a powerful tool that can keep you on track. Focus on your health goals, keep reminding yourself why you set out to do this, and envision the results. Here's how in seven steps.

1 QUIT THE EXCUSES

In this book, we have outlined everything you need to know and also worked hard to make sure some of your favorite foods can be replaced with tasty, healthful alternatives so you won't feel deprived. Making the right choices should be a piece of cake from now on, so you have no excuse!

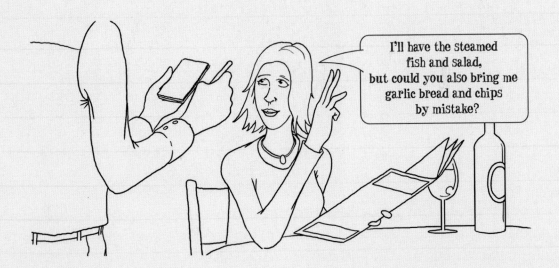

> I'll have the steamed fish and salad, but could you also bring me garlic bread and chips by mistake?

2 ACKNOWLEDGE THAT THIS IS NOT A "DIET"

... it's a lifestyle. Our bodies were not designed for liquid diets or frozen microwave meals based on points, which is why people often gain the weight back when they return to eating "normally." The changes we recommend are something you should consider implementing for the rest of your life. That might sound a bit scary, but it really isn't. Once you get the hang of it, it's easy. You get to eat really tasty food, and you'll look great for it! What's not to love about that?

3 REALIZE THAT HEALTHY FOOD DOES NOT MEAN BLAND AND BORING

Adapting your food intake is part and parcel of any new health plan, but that doesn't mean it's necessary to remove all taste and enjoyment from every eating occasion. If you don't enjoy what you eat, the chances of your sticking to it are incredibly slim. Our *Paleo Primer* recipes will make you realize that wholesome, nutrient-dense food can also be quite tasty!

What many people perceive as "healthy"

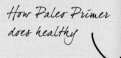

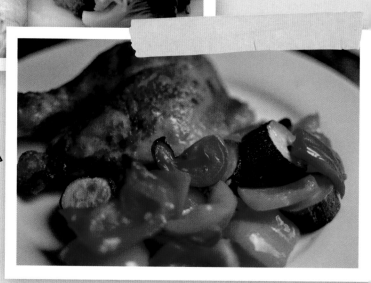

How Paleo Primer does healthy

4 KNOW THAT YOU CAN'T AFFORD NOT TO DO THIS

There's a perception that healthy food is time-consuming and expensive! It might be tempting to grab convenience foods on your way home because it's cheaper and quicker than investing in some high-quality meat, eggs, fish, or fresh vegetables. Yet understand that ultimately you will pay for it later—poor health can get pretty expensive! For those following a budget, check out *The Paleo Diet Budget Grocery Shopping Guide* available as an ebook download on RobbWolf.com.

5 LOVE THAT YOU CAN STILL HAVE A SOCIAL LIFE

People often perceive dieting and healthy living to mean the end of their social lives. This might be the case if you were following the maple syrup detox, as we doubt it is offered on any menu. Fortunately, you will find steak and spinach at most restaurants. It's incredibly easy to take our basic principles along on any night out. In Chapter 6, we also provide some guidance regarding the biggest challenge most people face during social occasions: alcohol! The key is moderation.

6 ACCEPT THAT YOU CAN LIVE WITHOUT PIZZA OR CAKE (BUT YOU DON'T HAVE TO!)

Everyone has an attachment to some favorite comfort foods, and going without can feel downright miserable. However, giving up these foods isn't always necessary; sometimes it's simply a matter of learning how to make healthier versions.

Chocolate Chestnut Fudge Cake (page 189)

Cauliflower Pizza (page 146)

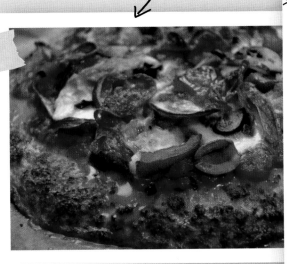

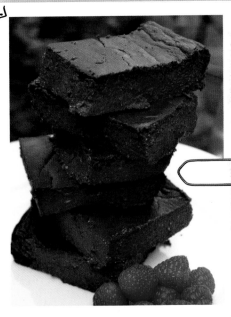

7 BELIEVE THAT YOU WILL SEE RESULTS!

Have patience; this isn't going to happen overnight. We work with many clients who have spent many years following a poor diet that has destroyed their health and metabolism, yet demand to see a six-pack within weeks. Have faith in your body, put good stuff into it, and you will get good stuff out ... yet understand that it may take time for your body to forgive you for all the years of abuse. The more you relax into your healthy routine and stop stressing about an inch here or there, the quicker things will happen.

CHAPTER 4

Nutrition -
Know Thy Stuff

I started [adopting paleo nutrition] with a friend at work, and we kept each other motivated and focused, comparing our homemade lunches in the office, discussing our evening meals and even going shopping together. I had never tried this kind of thing before, and it was surprisingly easy and enjoyable. **MARK SMITH** (Client)

The more you know about nutrition, the more control you will have over your health and destiny. So sit back, kick up your feet, and enjoy our guide on the basic principles.

NUTRIENTS IN SHORT

The human diet consists of two types of nutrients: *macronutrients* and *micronutrients.* The former provides the body with calories—or energy—and are found in three forms: carbohydrate, protein, and fat. The latter are compounds essential to human health and what you may know as vitamins, minerals, and antioxidants.

MACRONUTRIENTS (ENERGY)

These are referred to as "macro" because our bodies need large amounts of these nutrients to fulfill all our energy needs, which include growth and metabolism. The choices you make regarding these can have a huge impact on your health. To fully understand the importance of macronutrients, here is a quick overview of how our bodies utilize them.

PROTEIN
Protein is vital for the human body; it's what you're made of! Meat, fish, dairy, and eggs are examples of primary sources of protein within the human diet. The body breaks down protein into amino acids, which are used to build and maintain all the tissues—skin, hair, nails, and muscles. Protein molecules also act as transport vehicles for other nutrients, taking them to where they are needed in the body. Ensuring you have adequate protein intake is crucial for overall health.

CARBOHYDRATES
Carbohydrates are a major source of energy to the body. They are the preferred fuel source for not only the brain, but for muscles working at medium-to-high intensity as well. The body breaks down all carbohydrates into single molecules of glucose. How a carbohydrate is categorized depends on how it affects blood sugar levels. Those that absorb quickly into the body are known as "simple" or "high glycemic," as they create a rapid rise of sugar in the bloodstream. Examples include sweets and processed foods like bagels and cereal. The rapid surge of energy these foods supply is typically followed by a sudden decline, known as a blood sugar crash. When this happens, you're left feeling hungry and craving more sugar.

Avoiding such peaks and valleys is one of the key aspects to keeping the body healthy. The majority of your carbohydrate intake should be from "complex" or "low glycemic" sources, which are metabolized at a much slower rate and provide a steady release of sugar into the bloodstream. Foods high in fiber, such as vegetables and sweet potato, have a low glycemic impact as the fiber slows down the release of the sugars.

FAT

Let's start by establishing an important point: **FAT DOES NOT MAKE YOU FAT!**

Fat is an essential part of the human diet and has been for 2.5 million years. This includes the oft-maligned saturated fat that we typically obtain from animal sources. Have you ever met someone feeling absolutely miserable on a low-fat diet? We have! (We've been there ourselves!) This happens because fat performs a number of important functions in the body. It is a source of caloric energy and is integral in the transportation of nutrients around the body, especially the fat-soluble vitamins A, D, E, and K. Without fat in the diet, these vitamins simply cannot be adequately absorbed.

Fact is, fat can play a vital role in weight loss. Yes, you read that right! But it's the type and quality of the fat that counts. *Dr. Atkins' Diet Revolution*, which advocated a high-fat, low-carbohydrate diet when it was published back in 1972, didn't quite develop the magic formula, but it did establish that sugar and refined carbohydrates were a couple of the biggest enemies to our waistlines, not fat as commonly believed.

As previously mentioned, the single most important aim of your nutrition should be to balance your blood sugar levels. Dietary fat helps you accomplish that by slowing down the release of nutrients into the bloodstream, so by all means, add a little olive oil or butter to your meals. This will help regulate your appetite and keep your energy levels consistent.

Fat also insulates the body, protects our organs and joints, and is involved in many important hormonal and metabolic functions. And it's vital to brain health. In fact, evolutionary biologists assert that animal fat was the catalyst for the development of complex brain function that allowed us to branch away from our mostly vegetarian ape cousins.

So the main issue with the typical modern diet is not fat, but the type we consume. The Primal/paleo message to consume saturated fats liberally, and to restrict polyunsaturated vegetable and seed oils, is in direct conflict with the conventional wisdom that has been dispensed for decades. As leading science journalist Gary Taubes presents in great detail in his book *Why We Get Fat,* there has been absolutely no scientific evidence ever presented to suggest that saturated fats are unhealthy. It is only in the presence of excessive carbohydrate intake and insulin production that saturated fats can turn problematic in the bloodstream.

MICRONUTRIENTS (VITAMINS & MINERALS)

Micronutrients are elements that cannot be produced by the body but are essential for multiple physiological functions and must be obtained through dietary sources. These include minerals like zinc, magnesium, potassium, and all the vitamins: A, B, C, D, E, and K.

Sadly, vitamin and mineral deficiencies are becoming increasingly common across the globe. Much of the blame can be pinned on industrialized farming methods—for example, large monoculture planting and the use of chemical pesticides, herbicides, and fungicides—that decrease minerals in the soil. Consequently, produce grown in such soil is significantly depleted of micronutrients, a problem further aggravated by the common practices of premature picking, extended warehousing, and transporting food hundreds, if not thousands, of miles before reaching the supermarket, much less our plates. In addition to this, many of the foods we commonly eat, such as bread, pasta, and cereals, contain compounds known as phytates that bind to minerals like zinc and magnesium, making them unavailable for absorption into the body.

Securing an optimal intake of micronutrients is essential for your metabolism, particularly since many nutrients work synergistically to promote health. Zinc, for example, is needed for the absorption of vitamin A, so a deficiency in zinc will soon lead to a deficiency in vitamin A.

THE PROBLEM WITH OUR NUTRIENT SOURCES

We have established how macronutrients and micronutrients provide the foundation of your nutrition. Now let's assess our modern-day intake of both these elements, starting with the macronutrients on My Plate, the United States Department of Agriculture's current dietary guidelines published in 2011.

MODERN DAY ENERGY INTAKE

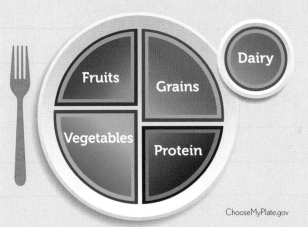

ChooseMyPlate.gov

As you can see, fruits (20 percent) and vegetables (30 percent) take up half the plate. OK, that's a fair enough start. Then we see manufactured foods, particularly those dense in processed carbohydrates, like bread and breakfast cereals (30 percent). Upon the advice of the US government, protein like soy, legumes, and lean and low-fat meat and fish provides a smaller contribution to overall caloric intake (20 percent). Americans are also advised to take in "fluid" dairy—that is, skim or low-fat 1% milk or calcium-fortified soy milk. Fats and oils are nowhere to be found on the plate, simply because the government considers them "empty calories," something that should be limited.

So, what's wrong with this low-fat picture? Simply put, we end up consuming excess carbohydrates. Over time, this taxes our bodies and causes us to lose our ability to process carbohydrates properly.

ENTER THE "MUFFIN TOP"

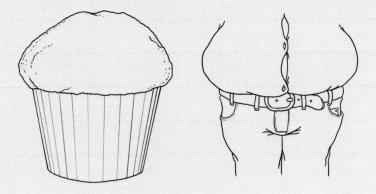

Fat storage around the middle is a good indicator that you are no longer using your carbohydrates for energy. The muffin top hasn't always plagued mankind, yet over the last few decades, man has certainly been fighting a losing battle with processed carbohydrates.

We are not in any way claiming that carbohydrates are "the enemy." Your carbohydrate demands vary significantly depending on factors such as your weight, activity levels, ethnicity, age, and general health. What we want to highlight is that there are better sources of carbohydrates, and they do not need to take up such a large portion of your plate. Featured on the opposite page is an improved plate created by Hannah Sutter, a former career lawyer and author of *Big Fat Lies: Is Your Government Making You Fat?*

On Sutter's plate there are no breads, pastas, couscous, cereals, crackers, bars, smoothies, cookies, or soft drinks. There is, however, plenty of protein and healthy fats. The results on the body speak for themselves.

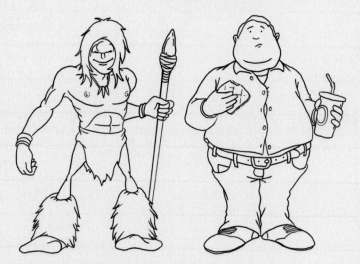

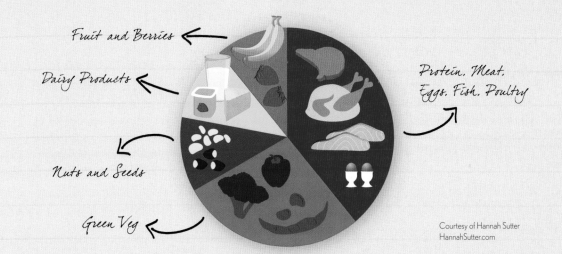

Fruit and Berries ←

Dairy Products ←

Nuts and Seeds

Green Veg ←

Protein, Meat,
Eggs, Fish, Poultry

Courtesy of Hannah Sutter
HannahSutter.com

HORMONES AND FAT STORAGE

Fat storage around the middle is also an indication that your body is losing its ability to respond to insulin, a hormone that is released when we eat. It instructs the body how to use carbohydrates and shuttles the sugar (glucose) into our cells for energy. If we eat heavily processed food, we experience high levels of sugar in the blood, prompting our bodies to produce large amounts of insulin to metabolize them. If this happens excessively, something known as insulin resistance can occur. When this happens, the cells in your body begin to tune out the constant presence of insulin. That means every time you eat, your cells will store glucose as fat instead of use it for energy.

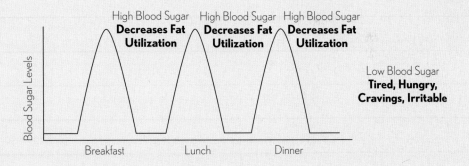

The solution is to balance your blood sugar levels with a healthy balance of fat, protein, and low glycemic carbohydrates. Together, they will provide the perfect combination for a slow, steady release of energy.

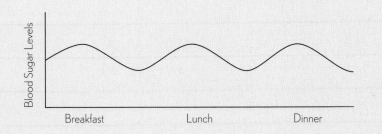

LEPTIN: THE OTHER HORMONE

Another hormone you should be aware of is leptin. In the 1990s, researchers at Rockefeller University established that leptin, which is actually stored in our fat cells, is the master hormone of body fat regulation. Interestingly, its role in the body dates back to our cavemen ancestors who endured times of famine. Leptin speaks to the brain and communicates whether the body has enough fat stores to make it through a period of starvation. If there aren't enough, the brain slows down the body's metabolic rate so that it will burn fewer calories throughout the day. Leptin also increases our appetites to motivate us to go out and find food. When we do finally eat, we receive a boost in the absorption of nutrients and rapidly increase fat stores in the body.

When leptin operates in a healthy fashion, it regulates body fat to optimal levels. However, a number of diet and lifestyle factors can cause "leptin resistance." When this occurs, leptin informs the brain that the body has enough fat stores—yet the brain is unable to comprehend the message. As a result, the brain continues to urge the body to store fat. Here are a few common factors that can cause leptin resistance.

- Excessive polyunsaturated fats (more on this coming up)
- Overeating and binge eating
- Calorie restriction
- Alcohol
- Wheat
- Fructose (more on this in Chapter 5)
- Stress
- Refined and processed carbohydrates
- Surges in insulin (as above)

OTHER MODERN FOODS EXPANDING OUR WAISTLINES

The advent of processed convenience foods ushered in a sharp decline in human health and physique. Clearly, sugary drinks, candy bars, french fries, ice cream, cakes, pastries, and chips haven't done us any good. Yet there's a lot more to the story than just junk food. Let's take a look.

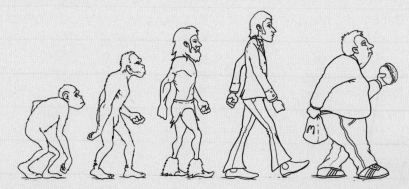

1. GRAINS

As discussed, public health recommendations in the US state that a large percentage of our energy should come from grain-based carbohydrates. This advice is given in the UK and other industrialized countries as well. Think about it: we start our day with breakfast cereal or toast, snack on crackers or cereal bars, have a sandwich for lunch, and our evening meal often includes a serving of pasta or bread.

This is problematic because gluten, the protein that gives dough its elasticity, is found in the grains that make up all these foods. Researchers estimate that as many as one-third of the US population is gluten intolerant or gluten insensitive, resulting in a multitude of negative reactions, including fatigue, joint pain, acid reflux, and skin problems. Far more serious is celiac disease, an immune reaction to gluten that causes damage to the lining of the small intestine and thus interferes with absorption of nutrients. Current research estimates that about 1 percent of the US population, or some 3 million people, have already been properly diagnosed with the disease. But most sufferers—an estimated 83 percent—don't even know they have the disease and are yet to be diagnosed. As public awareness increases, however, the number of celiac diagnoses are likely to dramatically increase over the next several years.[10]

Even the so-called "healthy" whole grains can be troublesome. As grains are seeds designed to grow into grasses, they contain mildly toxic substances that help protect them from being digested. Lectins, for example, are sticky proteins that bind to the lining of our guts, wreaking all sorts of havoc. If you have ever experienced gas, diarrhea, nausea, or bloating after consuming legumes or grains, you have experienced the wrath of lectins.

Phytates are another substance contained in grains. They bind to essential nutrients such as zinc, calcium, and magnesium, making it difficult for your body to absorb the minerals. As Mark Sisson points out in his seminal book *The Primal Blueprint*, unprocessed whole grains are typically the highest in phytates and interfere with vitamin D absorption and play a role in vitamin A, C, and B^{12} deficiencies.[11] That means that the whole grain products claimed to be high in nutrients are more likely leaving you nutrient deficient.

Research biochemist Robb Wolf, author of *The Paleo Solution*, provides a great summary of why all grains can be problematic for some people:

> Grains include anti-nutrients such as phytates, lectins, and immunoreactive protein. Lectins found in grains can damage the gut lining, which increases inflammation and is a discovered feature of autoimmune disease, insulin resistance, and liver pathology. All grains contain similar proteins to gluten, for instance oats have avenin, corn has zein, and rice has orzenin. What all these proteins have in common is a high content of the amino acid proline. Proline makes these proteins difficult to break down via normal digestion and they appear to have negative effects on the gut lining and overall health.[12]

---

[10] National Foundation for Celiac Awareness, www.celiaccentral.org/celiac-disease/facts-and-figures/
[11] Sisson, M., *Primal Blueprint*. Malibu, California: Primal Nutrition, Inc. 2009
[12] Wolf, R., *The Paleo Solution: The Original Human Diet United States*. Las Vegas, Nevada: Victory Belt Publishing, 2010

2. LOW FAT, FAT FREE, AND SUGAR FREE

Our Paleolithic ancestors thrived on large amounts of animal fats, oily fish, nuts, and seeds without issue. But today, fat has pretty much taken the blame for all the degenerative diseases we've experienced over the last few decades, with a billion dollar diet industry fueling the phobia. Thanks in no small part to the fat-free revolution, fat-free and low-fat options exist for just about every food item out there—even those that are inherently fattening (fat-free mayonnaise, anyone?). But have you ever wondered what takes the place of that removed fat? Answer: heaps of synthetic, non-food chemicals that wreak havoc on our metabolism and digestion. What's more, most low-fat and fat-free products contain loads of sugar or artificial sweeteners to make up for the lack of taste.

WHEN YOU SEE **FAT FREE** AND LOW FAT THINK **" CHEMICAL SHIT STORM "**

Artificial sweeteners are a beast unto themselves. Heralded as "the weight-loss solution," these fake sweeteners actually increase appetite levels and elevate our desire for more sweet stuff.[13] Sweeteners known as sugar alcohols are incompletely absorbed in the digestive tract (so they do not cause a rise in blood sugar levels), but they tend to ferment in the bowel and may cause excessive wind, bloating, and diarrhea.[14]

And if all that isn't enough to put you off, research is investigating the potential neurotoxic effect of artificial sweeteners and associations with conditions like dementia, Alzheimer's disease, and Parkinson's disease. For more information, read *Dying for a Diet Coke*, a free report put together by Emory University.[15]

3. ADDITIVES, PRESERVATIVES, THICKENERS, GUMS, AND STABILIZERS

The food industry has become ever more creative in finding substances to preserve, bind, thicken, and stabilize their products. These substances are ubiquitous in prepackaged foods like ready-made meals, chips, condiments, dressings, candy bars, cookies, and desserts, and can be incredibly aggressive on the digestive system. Many people are sensitive to these substances and experience mild reactions after eating particular foods. One example is sulfites, used in the preservation of wine and dried fruits. They commonly cause digestive problems or a flare-up on the skin.

4. COMMERCIAL DAIRY

Including or excluding dairy in your diet is an individual decision. Some nutritionists strongly argue that adults should not be consuming milk-based products because we lose the ability to digest the sugar (lactose) in milk at an early age when our bodies stop producing lactase enzymes. Some experts have

[13] M. Tordoff, A. Alleva. "Oral stimulation with aspartame increases hunger." *Physiological Behavior* 47.3 (1990): 555-559.
[14] P. Gibson, S. Shepherd. "Evidence-based dietary management of functional gastrointestinal symptoms: The FODMAP approach." *Journal of Gastroenterology and Hepatology* 25.2 (2010) 252-258. S. Proctor, D. Vine, Y. Wang, M. Jacome-Sosa. "Beneficial effects of vaccenic acid on postprandial lipid metabolism and dyslipidemia: Impact of natural trans-fats to improve CVD risk." *Lipid Technology* 22.5 (2010): 103-106.
[15] C. Wheeler. "Dying for a Diet Coke," http://rense.com/general78/dying.htm

voiced concerns about the growth factors and hormones in milk and their potential to promote the development of certain cancers.[16] Other studies link dairy with autoimmune conditions like inflammatory bowel disease,[17] rheumatoid arthritis,[18] and multiple sclerosis.[19] If you have health concerns you wish to resolve, it is worthwhile to remove dairy products for a period of time to see if your symptoms improve.

But like fat, not all dairy is equal. Dairy products from grass-fed cows, sheep, and goats can provide an excellent source of vitamins, minerals, and essential fats. Grass-fed dairy products that consist predominantly of fat—for example, heavy cream and butter—are low in lactose and contain vitamins A, D, E, and K. They also contain a healthy fat known as conjugated linoleic acid (CLA), which has been found to have anti-cancer properties.[20] Ghee, which is clarified butter, has no lactose in it and is great to use for cooking if you are lactose intolerant.

So while some dairy products do in fact provide health benefits, they too have suffered at the hands of the food industry. Commercial dairy now has most of its healthy components like saturated fat, beneficial bacteria, and enzymes removed. The skimming and pasteurization process results in a higher sugar (lactose) content, fewer nutrients, and a dairy product that is almost impossible to digest effectively. In Chapter 8, we'll detail some highly nutritious sources of dairy to add to your shopping cart. In the meantime, aim to at least limit your consumption of commercial dairy products, as these are subjected to a number of chemical processes that remove most of the nutritional goodness, especially in these products:

※ Skimmed, semi-skimmed, and whole homogenized milk

※ UHT milk (Ultra High Temperature processing for prolonged shelf life)

※ Cream substitutes

※ Low-fat or processed cheeses

※ Low-fat spreads or margarines

5. POLYUNSATURATED VEGETABLE OILS AND HYDROGENATED TRANS FATS

Trans fats are increasingly receiving recognition for their harmful effects on the body and have been implicated in the progression of heart disease, cancer, and diabetes. Again, not all fats are equal. There is a very clear distinction between naturally occurring trans fats (like those found in meat and dairy products) and trans fats made through the chemical treatment of vegetable fats (known as hydrogenation).

Naturally occurring trans fats in meat and dairy have a beneficial effect and lower many of the risk factors for cardiovascular disease.[21] Hydrogenated trans fats (also called partially hydrogenated oils), on the other hand, provide zero health benefits. These fake fats were developed to keep solid at room temperature and increase the shelf life of products like cakes, sweets, cookies, fried foods, and prepackaged meals. It is worth noting that partially hydrogenated oils are used in many restaurants and

[16] J. Plant. *Your Life In Your Hands: Understanding, Preventing and Overcoming Breast Cancer.* London: Virgin Books (2011).
[17] A. Lerner, T. Rossi, B. Park, B. Albini, E. Lebenthal. "Serum antibodies to cow's milk proteins in pediatric inflammatory bowel disease. Crohn's disease versus ulcerative colitis." *Acta Paediatrica Scandinavica* 78.3 (1989): 384-89.
[18] J. Kjeldsen-Kragh, M. Hvatum, M. Haugen, O. Førre, H. Scott. "Antibodies against dietary antigens in rheumatoid arthritis patients treated with fasting and a one-year vegetarian diet." *Clinical and Experimental Rheumatology* 13.2 (1995):167-72.
[19] D. Malosse, H. Perron, A. Sasco, J. Seigneurin. "Correlation between milk and dairy product consumption and multiple sclerosis prevalence: a worldwide study." *Neuroepidemiology* 11.4-6 (1992): 304-12.
[20] C. Larsson, L. Bergkvist, A. Wolk. "High-fat dairy food and conjugated linoleic acid intakes in relation to colorectal cancer incidence in the Swedish Mammography Cohort." *American Journal of Clinical Nutrition* 82.4 (2005): 894-900
[21] S. Proctor et al. *Lipid Technology* 22.5 (2010): 103-106.

fast food outlets, though some places, like New York City, have banned the fat altogether. Increasingly—and thankfully—hydrogenated trans fats are being removed from many foods due to a strong association with incidents of disease.[22]

Then there are the polyunsaturated fatty acids (PUFAs), which include the essential fatty acids omega-3 and omega-6. These fats are termed "essential" because our bodies cannot produce them and so they must be obtained from our diet. But unlike saturated animal fats, polyunsaturated fats do not include hydrogen atoms, which makes them unstable and prone to oxidation. This is why it is imperative that omega-3 and omega-6 fats are sourced and consumed as fresh as possible. And they should be consumed in equal measure.

This is the how humans in prehistoric times consumed these fats, and, as we've learned, they did not suffer from obesity or inflammatory diseases.[23] Today, however, omega-6 fats (sourced from nuts, seeds, and some vegetables) predominate over omega-3 fats (sourced from fatty fish, grass-fed meats, eggs, and some nuts) in the typical modern diet—by about twenty to one! And for some people, even higher than that! Fact is, a disproportionate amount of our modern fats are sourced from vegetable and seed oils (typically corn, canola, soybean, sunflower, and safflower), and are usually consumed as low-fat spreads and cooking oils. Despite the "heart healthy" image of these processed omega-6 fats, they are now recognized as one of the primary culprits in the development of chronic disease. We see a prevalence of omega-6 fats in packaged foods such as donuts, cookies, and ready-made meals, but also in low-fat vegetable spreads and salad oils. They're even seen in the fat of animals raised on corn, soy, and other grains. (Yep, grains are bad for farm animals, too!) We'll discuss the virtues of grass-fed meat in Chapter 8, but the main take-away message for now is to reduce the omega-6 fats in your diet and increase the omega-3s.

UNDOING THE DAMAGE: TRANSFORMING YOUR PLATE

Years of eating modern-day foods have left many of us struggling with digestive issues, nutrient deficiency, blood sugar imbalance, and inflammation. So here's the plan: to start fixing your body, strive to do the following in your diet.

✴ BALANCE BLOOD SUGAR LEVELS
To slow down the release of sugar after meals, increase healthy fats and protein alongside the right choice of carbohydrates on your plate.

✴ LIMIT OMEGA-6 FATS AND CONSUME MORE OMEGA-3 FATS
Cavemen consumed equal amounts of omega-3 and omega-6 and didn't suffer from the inflammatory diseases that we do today. The key is to decrease your intake of grains and polyunsaturated oils that are high in omega-6, and eat lots more omega-3 foods such as oily fish, egg yolks, and grass-fed meats.

✴ AVOID FOOD TOXINS
To support your digestion, metabolism, and maximum absorption of nutrients, avoid foods that contain gluten, lectins, phytates, and all synthetic non-foods like sweeteners and chemical preservatives.

- - - - - - - - - - - - - - - -

[22] F. Kummerow. "The negative effects of hydrogenated trans fats and what to do about them. Atherosclerosis." 205.2 (2009):458-65
[23] A. Simopoulos. "Evolutionary aspects of diet, the omega-6/omega-3 ratio and genetic variation: nutritional implications for chronic diseases." *Biomedicine & Pharmacotherapy* 60 (2006): 502-507

✳ BOOST MICRONUTRIENTS (VITAMINS AND MINERALS)

Every time you eat, make sure your plate is packed with nutrients. For example, swap your bread and pasta for a serving of sweet potatoes and roasted vegetables. This will more than double the dose of vitamins and minerals on your plate. Check out this comparison of vitamins and minerals in a serving of sweet potato versus a serving of pasta on the opposite page.

one serving of cooked sweet potato

Vitamins

Amounts Per Selected Serving		%DV
Vitamin A	38433 IU	769%
Vitamin C	39.2 mg	65%
Vitamin D	-	-
Vitamin E (Alpha Tocopherol)	1.4 mg	7%
Vitamin K	4.6 mcg	6%
Thiamin	0.2 mg	14%
Riboflavin	0.2 mg	12%
Niacin	3.0 mg	15%
Vitamin B6	0.6 mg	29%
Folate	12.0 mcg	3%
Vitamin B12	0.0 mcg	0%
Pantothenic Acid	1.8 mg	18%
Choline	26.2 mg	-
Betaine	69.2 mg	-

Minerals

Amounts Per Selected Serving		%DV
Calcium	76.0 mg	8%
Iron	1.4 mg	8%
Magnesium	54.0 mg	14%
Phosphorus	108 mg	11%
Potassium	950 mg	27%
Sodium	72.0 mg	3%
Zinc	0.6 mg	4%
Copper	0.3 mg	16%
Manganese	1.0 mg	50%
Selenium	0.4 mcg	1%
Fluoride	-	-

one serving of cooked pasta

Vitamins

Amounts Per Selected Serving		%DV
Vitamin A	11.4 IU	0%
Vitamin C	0.0 mg	0%
Vitamin D	-	-
Vitamin E (Alpha Tocopherol)	-	-
Vitamin K	-	-
Thiamin	0.1 mg	8%
Riboflavin	0.1 mg	5%
Niacin	0.6 mg	3%
Vitamin B6	0.0 mg	1%
Folate	35.5 mcg	9%
Vitamin B12	0.1 mcg	1%
Pantothenic Acid	0.1 mg	1%
Choline	-	-
Betaine	-	-

Minerals

Amounts Per Selected Serving		%DV
Calcium	3.4 mg	0%
Iron	0.6 mg	4%
Magnesium	10.3 mg	3%
Phosphorus	35.9 mg	4%
Potassium	13.7 mg	0%
Sodium	3.4 mg	0%
Zinc	0.3 mg	2%
Copper	0.1 mg	3%
Manganese	0.1 mg	6%
Selenium	-	-

Source: Nutrition Data

THE A TO ZINC GUIDE TO MICRONUTRIENTS

Food is the best source for vitamins and minerals. Here's a guide to ensure you get your daily dose.

VITAMIN A
carrots, spinach, sweet peppers, parsley, liver, sweet potato, cayenne pepper, apricots, asparagus, butternut squash

B VITAMINS
beef, turkey, salmon, sardines, tuna, liver, bananas, lentils, chicken, spinach, avocado

VITAMIN C
cauliflower, parsley, broccoli, strawberries, lemon juice, sweet peppers, raspberries, celery, zucchini

VITAMIN D
shrimp, prawns, sardines, cod, eggs, sunlight (NOTE: Sunlight is really the best source of this nutrient, providing up to ten times more than dietary sources.)

VITAMIN E
almonds, Swiss chard, spinach, olives, blueberries

VITAMIN K1
parsley, kale, spinach, Swiss chard, collard greens, basil, broccoli, cabbage

VITAMIN K2
egg yolks, organ meats, grass-fed butter

CALCIUM
spinach, collard greens, basil, cinnamon, yogurt, Swiss chard, kale, milk, goat milk

COPPER
calf's liver, portobello mushrooms, spinach, cashews, kale, eggplant, sesame seeds, zucchini

IODINE
sea vegetables, yogurt, eggs, strawberries

IRON
spinach, turmeric, basil, cinnamon, green beans, shiitake mushrooms, Swiss chard, venison, asparagus

MAGNESIUM
spinach, Swiss chard, pumpkin seeds, broccoli, cucumber, flaxseed

POTASSIUM
portobello mushrooms, Swiss chard, celery, butternut squash, bananas

SELENIUM
Brazil nuts, cod, shiitake mushrooms, tuna, shrimp, prawns, sardines, salmon

ZINC
calf's liver, oysters, portobello mushrooms, spinach, grass-fed beef, lamb, zucchini, venison, pumpkin seeds, sesame seeds

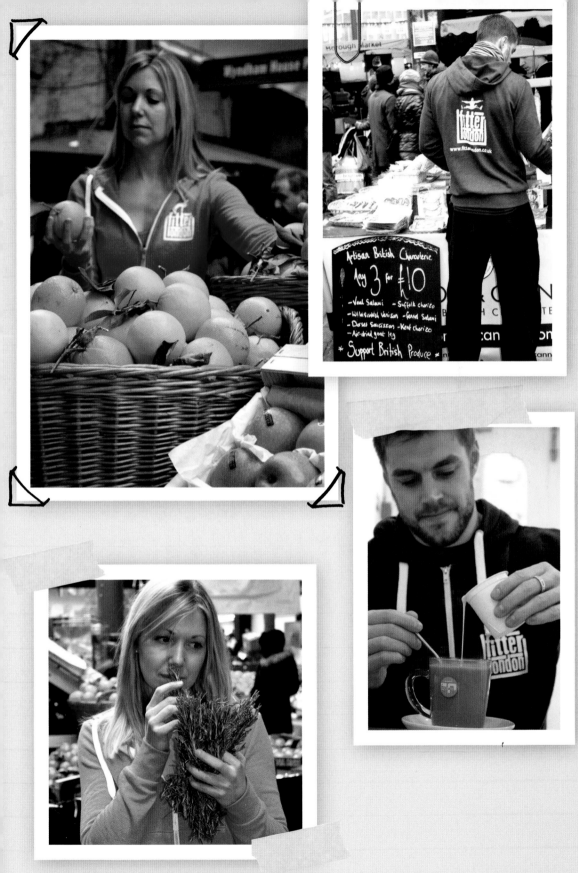

CHAPTER 5

REMOVING SUGAR, GRAINS, AND LEGUMES

> **❝** The last six months of eating right has had a more positive effect on my body than almost ten years of training. I've finally realized that you can train as much as you like, but if you put crap into your body, you'll get crap out of it. **ROB JORDAN** (Client) **❞**

Removing grains, legumes, and sugar from your diet can be challenging. This chapter will help you understand where they are found, why you should avoid some more than others, and how you can replace them.

THE SWEET STUFF

One thing you probably don't need to hear from us is that sugar is evil. It suppresses the immune system,[24] disrupts hormones that regulate our appetite,[25] fuels the growth of cancer cells,[26] encourages fat storage and weight gain ... surely you don't need much more convincing to limit the sweet stuff as much as possible!

One sugar we should all aim to avoid is fructose syrup, or high fructose corn syrup (HFCS) as it is commonly labeled on many processed foods. This substance has been linked to several metabolic disorders by negatively affecting the hormones that regulate appetite and body fat.[27] Foods containing this sugar tend to be confectionary and include sweets, chips, cookies, and soft drinks. Motto of the story: always check the label!

We know there may be special occasions where a dessert is called for, so we have put together some healthier versions of traditional treats like cakes, cookies, and puddings. In our dessert recipes, we use a combination of fruits like berries, bananas, apples, and dried apricots or coconut sugar. We also use raw honey. Even though it contains some fructose, it has less impact on our blood sugar levels than processed honey, and you only need a small amount. We selected these because they are all low-glycemic sweeteners and provide additional nutritional benefits in the form of antioxidants, vitamins, and minerals.

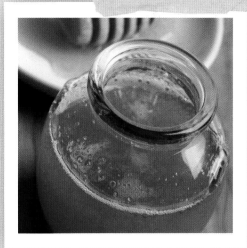

[24] A. Sanchez, J. Reeser, H. Lau, P. Yahiku, R. Willard, P. Mcmillan, S. Cho, A. Magie. "Role of sugars in human neutrophilic phagocytosis." *American Journal of Clinical Nutrition* 26.11 (1973): 1180-1184.

[25] S. Roberts. "High-glycemic index foods, hunger, and obesity: is there a connection?" *Nutrition Review* 58 (2000): 163-169

[26] S. Seeley. "Diet and breast cancer: the possible connection with sugar consumption." *Medical Hypotheses* 11.3 (1983): 319-27.

[27] L. Tappy and K. Anne-Le. "Metabolic Effects of Fructose and the Worldwide Increase in Obesity." *Physiological Reviews* 90 (2010): 23-46.

GOING AGAINST THE GRAIN

Now that we understand how gluten, phytates, and lectins can harm our health, it is vital to single out the most offending grains that contain them.

TYPICAL GRAINS INCLUDE:

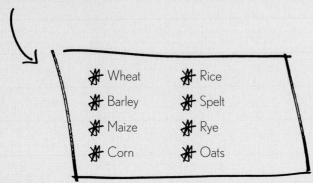

* Wheat
* Barley
* Maize
* Corn
* Rice
* Spelt
* Rye
* Oats

WHERE FOUND:
Bread, pasta, rice, couscous, cookies, cakes, breadsticks, cereals, crackers, sauces, condiments, and confections. They are often hidden in many other foods, so again, always check labels.

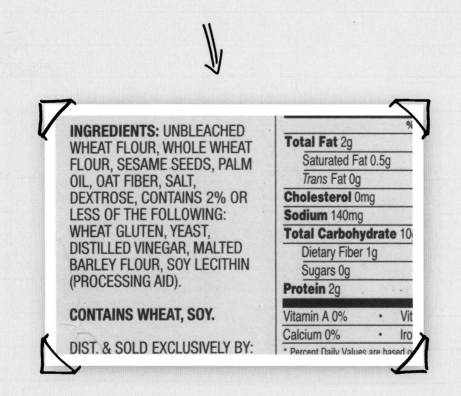

INGREDIENTS: UNBLEACHED WHEAT FLOUR, WHOLE WHEAT FLOUR, SESAME SEEDS, PALM OIL, OAT FIBER, SALT, DEXTROSE, CONTAINS 2% OR LESS OF THE FOLLOWING: WHEAT GLUTEN, YEAST, DISTILLED VINEGAR, MALTED BARLEY FLOUR, SOY LECITHIN (PROCESSING AID).

CONTAINS WHEAT, SOY.

DIST. & SOLD EXCLUSIVELY BY:

	%
Total Fat 2g	
Saturated Fat 0.5g	
Trans Fat 0g	
Cholesterol 0mg	
Sodium 140mg	
Total Carbohydrate 10g	
Dietary Fiber 1g	
Sugars 0g	
Protein 2g	
Vitamin A 0% • Vit	
Calcium 0% • Iro	
* Percent Daily Values are based on	

REPLACING GRAINS

So, if not pasta, what else can you fill your plate with? As we've mentioned throughout this book, to make sure you get a daily dose of vitamins and minerals, vegetables should absolutely dominate. Also, some starch-based foods do not contain as many anti-nutrients, and so do not cause problems for most people.

OPTION 1: VEGETABLES
Vegetables are, of course, one of the best options; sometimes you just need a little inspiration. Check out the following.

Cauliflower Rice (page 154)

Vegetable Spaghetti (page 160)

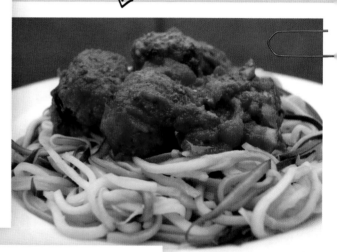

Butternut Smash (page 157)

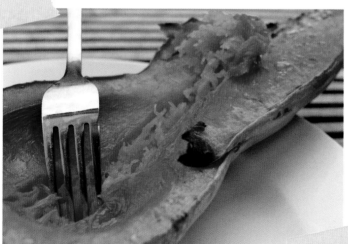

OPTION 2: SAFE STARCHES

"Safe starches" is a term coined by *Perfect Health Diet* authors Paul Jaminet and Shou-Ching Shih Jaminet to convey the idea that some dietary carbohydrates can be consumed with minimal health risks and maximum nutritional benefits. That is, most people can enjoy safe starches without the digestive and immune compromising effects they might otherwise experience with grains and sugars.

Some of our favorite sources of safe starches include sweet potato, plantains, and white rice. Although white rice is a grain, it is gluten-free and low in phytates. If prepared properly (rinsed, soaked, and boiled), it is easier to digest and can usually be tolerated by most people. White is preferential to brown as removing the whole grain means it is less likely to hinder the absorption of vitamins and minerals. Refer to the following graphical representation from the Jaminet's *Perfect Health Diet* for the recommended consumption levels in various food categories. *Note*: The amounts represented on the graph (for example, 1 pound per day) convey the total precooked weight of the food, most of which is water.

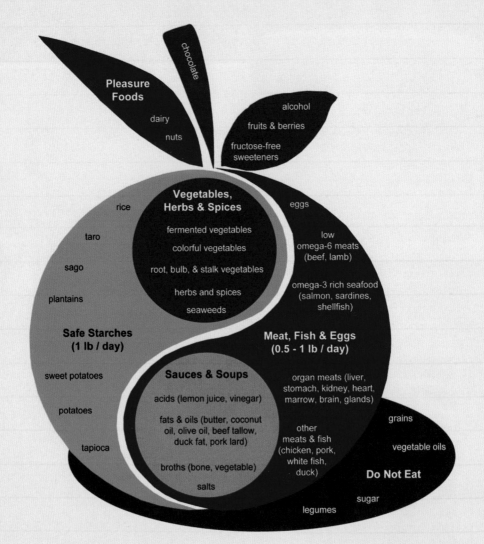

© www.PerfectHealthDiet.com

TO BEAN OR NOT TO BEAN

Legumes (often known as pulses or beans) are often perceived as a healthy choice due to their high fiber content. However, they contain similar anti-nutrients to grains (lectins and phytates), which, as we've discussed, can cause health issues for some people.

Legumes are often favored as a source of dietary protein, but they are not particularly a dense source compared to meat, fish, shellfish, or eggs as they contain more carbohydrate than protein. Many people also eat legumes to boost vitamin and mineral intake, but since they contain phytates, these nutrients are often poorly absorbed. Vegetables provide a much more efficient source.

And let's not forget the fart factor! The carbohydrates in legumes are often not fully digested and do not get properly absorbed in the gut. The bacteria in the digestive system then ferment these carbohydrates, creating wind and bloating. This can also potentially upset the balance of bacteria in your gut by feeding bad bacteria, which may lead to chronic digestive disorders.

LEGUMES

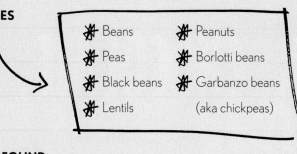

- Beans
- Peas
- Black beans
- Lentils
- Peanuts
- Borlotti beans
- Garbanzo beans
  (aka chickpeas)

WHERE FOUND:
Hummus, baked beans, dhal, ready-made meals, and packaged salads.

TWO BEANS WE DON'T MIND OCCASIONALLY
There are two beans we eat on occasion: **green beans** and **green peas**. Although still classified as legumes, if these beans are consumed fresh and cooked well, the anti-nutrient content is significantly lowered. Also, these are commonly offered when eating out and certainly make a better side dish than bread or pasta.

TWO BEANS WE ALWAYS AVOID
Soybeans have a reputation as a healthy dietary choice. Yet many of the soy products we consume—soy milk, soy yogurt, and soy cheeses—are industrially processed. They bare little resemblance to tempeh, miso, and natto, the fermented soy dishes used in ancient Asian traditions.

The truth is, all soy contains compounds called isoflavones, a phytoestrogen that acts like the female reproductive hormone estrogen. Although marketed as helpful for women experiencing menopause, evidence suggests that soy can adversely affect thyroid function in both men and women.

Peanuts are in fact legumes and are incredibly high in omega-6 fats, with two handfuls providing around 11 grams. Remember this is the fat we wish to limit. Peanuts also contain a mold known as aflatoxin, which has been shown to increase the risk of liver cancer.

CHAPTER 6

CAFFEINE, CHOCOLATE, AND ALCOHOL

> **❝** I was determined to get a six-pack, but equally extremely attached to lattes, chocolate brownies, and few too many drinks on the weekend. So I gave these habits up for a month. It really taught me how to appreciate these pleasures in life again. Moderation is the key; a few squares of dark chocolate and a couple of glasses of quality red wine. Now I have a little of something I enjoy AND a six-pack ... perfect! **MANRAJ ARORA** (Client) **❞**

We had to devote a whole chapter to these three "can't live withouts," because almost every client has an attachment to at least one of them. We point out our clients, but we actually mean *we* can't live without them either! The good news is there are some health benefits to consuming these—you just need to know how to make better choices.

CAFFEINE: COFFEE

Coffee for us is a bit of a nonnegotiable. We just love the stuff! Still, too many of us have transformed our daily cup of joe into a vente triple-shot latte.

But maybe that's good news: a number of studies suggest that moderate coffee consumption can provide health benefits. For one, coffee is rich in antioxidant compounds. It has also been shown to improve cognitive function, alleviate constipation, and protect against cardiovascular disease.

Now the bad news: contrasting studies list potential negative impacts, including decreased insulin sensitivity and an increased diuretic effect. Coffee has also been shown to exacerbate ulcers, irritable bowel syndrome, gastritis, and other such gastrointestinal disorders. The majority of research focusing on these negative impacts cite caffeine as the culprit. Indeed, a regular cup of coffee contains around 100 to 200 mg of caffeine, which is known to stimulate the release of cortisol (our bodies' stress hormone). If we consume too much caffeine throughout the day, we risk chronically elevating our cortisol levels. In the long term, this can lead to weight gain, sleep troubles, and a depressed immune system.

It's always best to remove all coffee if you are feeling stressed, as the caffeine can heighten the symptoms. Try switching to a naturally decaffeinated coffee or a Swiss water processed brew instead. Unlike conventional decafs, these contain none of the chemical solvents that are typically used to remove the caffeine from the coffee beans.

《 TIP 》 Add heavy whipping cream, half and half, or a teaspoon of coconut oil to your coffee—the fat slows down the impact of the caffeine on your blood sugar level. We carry a small container of heavy cream with us whenever we visit our favorite coffee shops. Coffee and cream beats a latte any day!

CAFFEINE: TEA

All types of tea are renowned for their health benefits. As a natural source of antioxidants, polyphenols, and flavonoids, tea can help prevent oxidation in the body by soaking up free radicals, the bad guys that contribute to rapid aging, cancer, and heart disease. Ideally, tea should be consumed without any milk or sugar to really benefit from the healthy compounds it contains.

 If you struggle taking black tea without milk, try white-leaf tea. It's much lighter and almost tastes like it has milk added! (We did say almost.)

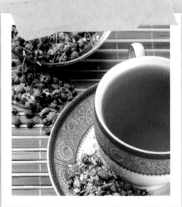

One issue with drinking too much tea is that it contains substances known as tannins, which can hinder your body's absorption of minerals, especially iron. As such, it's a good idea to avoid drinking it near mealtimes. Another issue, similar to that of coffee, is the caffeine content. Herbal infusion teas such as peppermint, ginger, and cinnamon are wonderful caffeine-free alternatives and an easy way to obtain nutrients that support your health objectives. Green tea provides exceptional health properties, including anti-cancer and fat-burning properties, improved blood sugar balance, and liver support. Aim to drink one or two cups a day if you can.

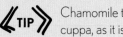 Chamomile tea makes the perfect after-dinner cuppa, as it is great for curbing sweet cravings and aiding relaxation.

CHOCOLATE

Chocolate—who doesn't love it, need it, want it? This is not surprising considering studies have shown that just a couple of squares are enough to elevate our "good mood" serotonin levels.

Chocolate contains two main ingredients: cocoa solids and butter from cocoa beans. If you have ever tried 100 percent cocoa, you'll understand why sugar and other flavors are typically added! Just make sure you consume chocolate that is at least 70 percent cocoa to receive the health benefits it has to offer. Dark chocolate is much lower in sugar than milk chocolate, and the bitter taste can help to counter-balance sugar cravings. It's also a rich source of antioxidants.

But beware: for some of us, sweet foods like chocolate (no matter how dark) can trigger more cravings for sugary foods. And despite containing loads of magnesium, calcium, and potassium, chocolate has high levels of phytates. As mentioned earlier, these can inhibit the absorption of beneficial minerals.

The best way to consume chocolate is to choose an organic, fair-trade brand, and enjoy a small 1-ounce serving rather than devouring an entire 3-ounce bar.

ALCOHOL

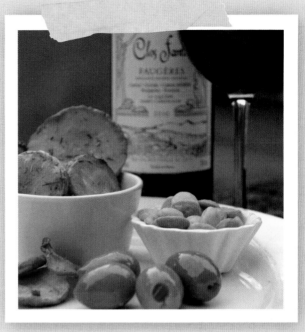

One of our biggest battles with clients is getting them to reduce their alcohol consumption. We often hear the phrase, "It's part of my job to wine and dine." But let's be honest: you aren't really paid to binge on booze! Alcohol will always be at odds with any health goal. It offers zero nutritional value and compromises fat metabolism. And if abused, it can lead to a number of health issues.

For one, alcohol is a toxin to the liver and taken in excess can lead to fatty liver disease. It also causes dehydration and headaches. (Can you say hangover?) Beer is especially problematic for many people as it contains gluten, which, as we have previously discussed, compromises healthy digestive and immune function. It also raises the body's estrogen levels, leading to fat storage in the legs and the abdomen. Cocktails and spirits mixed with soft drinks should be avoided due to their high sugar content as alcohol tends to accelerate the conversion of sugar into fat. But it's not just the sugary cocktails. Alcohol in any form depletes the body's vitamin B stores and speeds up the transit time of our food through the gut, hindering the absorption of nutrients. Alcohol also rapidly lowers blood sugar levels in the body, which can cause fatigue and disrupt sleep.

But worry not. We're not going to suggest that you become a teetotaler. We only ask that you incorporate your libations sensibly into your healthy lifestyle. In other words, use it in moderation. When used wisely, alcohol consumption can actually have some beneficial effects. It often helps people to relax, and some studies have also demonstrated an association between moderate alcohol consumption and a lower risk of heart disease. Keeping alcohol consumption low and limiting it to special occasions is usually best. Wines are considered a marginally better choice as they contain slightly less alcohol and provide a source of antioxidants.

Sensible drinking is a highly individual issue with serious implications to consider. While we often make recommendations to individual clients to limit their consumption on social occasions to two servings (one serving being a 5-ounce glass of wine, an 8-ounce glass of beer, or a cocktail consisting of 1.5 ounces of spirit mixed with soda water), body weight and other variables can create extreme disparity here. Striving to keep up with your mates in the weight room is fine, but it's best for you to regulate your alcohol intake individually to avoid impairment and maximize the enjoyment of your beverages and your socializing. And of course, if you find yourself unable to control your drinking, it's better to refrain from drinking altogether.

 Seek out organic and biodynamic wines and craft beers that help lessen the chemical load on the liver.

CHAPTER 7
Getting Started

Now that you have all the information you need, here are some practical first steps to help get you going.

EAT REGULAR MEALS

The first thing to do is get into the habit of eating regular meals. Set yourself up for the day by eating a breakfast high in protein and fat as this will help stabilize blood sugar levels. Also ensure that you eat a small meal every three or four hours to help develop consistent energy levels. This could be a simple snack such as a boiled egg, half an avocado, or a homemade burger. After a few weeks, once you notice your appetite stabilize considerably, you can start to experiment with your meal frequency. Some people prefer to have just two meals a day, others like to have more. It really depends on your activity levels, age, and routine. Learn to listen to your body—it will usually tell you what it needs.

HOW MUCH?
So what exactly is the magic ratio of protein, fat, and carbohydrate? The truth of the matter is, the only person who can really establish this is you. Your macronutrient requirements vary depending upon your activity levels, age, body composition, stress levels, and health conditions.

Start by following our advice on portion control on the next page. Ideally, after a meal you should feel satiated and your energy levels should remain relatively consistent. You should be able to stay active on a daily basis, feel positive, and have enough fuel in the tank to support your exercise regimen. You should be able to last three to five hours between meals without even thinking about food. If you do find yourself hungry or excessively tired or light-headed, you may need to adjust your intake. Ensure that you are hitting your minimal protein requirements across your meals first (see page 46), and then begin to increase your intake of healthy fats and carbohydrates.

CARBOHYDRATES

By swapping out grains and legumes for vegetables, the caveman style of eating is naturally lower in carbohydrates. You may wish to adjust this according to your own health goals. For instance, if you are storing excess body fat, reducing your carbohydrate consumption initially may help you reach your weight-loss goals. Without carbohydrates, the body will start to use fat for energy; this is known as becoming "fat adapted." Mark Sisson provides a great overview of this in his book *The Primal Blueprint*. The carb curve opposite is taken from the book and illustrates how to adapt your carbohydrates to your body composition. If

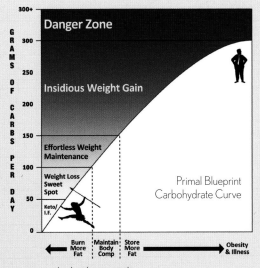

you are looking for rapid weight loss, you can try reducing your carbohydrate intake to 50 grams a day. Many people see weight loss occur in the region of 100 grams of carbohydrates a day. If you are decreasing your carbohydrates significantly, you may wish to increase your intake of healthy fats, as ingested dietary fat and stored body fat will now become the main sources of energy that your body will burn. There are many online nutrient calculators that can help you establish what 50 to 100 grams of carbohydrates may look like. We use CronoMeter.com and FitDay.com.

If you lead a physically active lifestyle that includes participating in a considerable amount of sports, strength training, or endurance exercise—and you maintain acceptable body fat levels—you may wish to consume larger quantities of carbohydrates than indicated on the Primal Blueprint Carbohydrate Curve. In this case, we recommend carbs like sweet potatoes because they have a high nutritional value and are absent of anti-nutrients. Extra servings of fruits, such as bananas and berries, work well, too. Or, if you follow the *Perfect Health Diet*, you may wish to include some white rice. One of the best times to consume carbohydrates is after exercising. This is when the cells within the body are more likely to respond to insulin as there is a greater need to replenish nutrients.

PROTEIN

Protein recommendations vary significantly from person to person. Base your intake on your body weight. The lowest recommendations are around 0.5 grams per pound of body weight (for the inactive), and at the higher end (for devoted fitness enthusiasts), around 1 gram per pound of body weight. If you are exercising regularly, stressed out, or working hard, your protein requirements can increase, so experiment with your intake. A fillet of meat or fish about the size of your fist yields between 20 to 25 grams.

FAT

If you are reducing your carbohydrates, a high fat intake will help maintain energy and satiety as well as support the reduction of body fat. Whether it's coconut oil in your coffee, butter on your green vegetables, olive oil drizzled over salads, avocados eaten straight out of their shell, or the fat found in grass-fed meat, monounsaturated and saturated fats can make up around 60 to 80 percent of your daily total caloric intake when you are truly Primal-aligned and grain and sugar free. Again, use an online nutrient calculator to experiment.

PORTION CONTROL

Portion control is a common obstacle we see with our clients, especially since our recipes are so tasty! But it's essential not to overeat. Portion control not only helps you manage your body composition but also encourages better digestion. Your plate should look something like this: A protein, such as fish, chicken, beef, or lamb, about the size of your fist. And two vegetables, each also about fist size. One vegetable should be green and the other can be more starchy, something like a sweet potato or butternut squash. Every meal should include some healthy fat, for example, a tablespoon of olive oil or butter over your vegetables.

Eat your meals slowly and in a relaxed environment, ideally not at your desk working or on the sofa watching TV. Take time to taste, smell, and enjoy your meals. This allows your brain to register that you have eaten and encourages a healthy balance between the hormones that stimulate your appetite and signal a sense of fullness. Also be sure to chew each bite thoroughly, ten to fifteen times, as breaking down food in the mouth is vital to healthy digestion.

A QUICK HEADS UP ON WITHDRAWALS AND CRAVINGS

Many processed foods are addictive. Food manufacturers have spent years researching the tastes and textures that we love and crave so they can fill their products with them. The first time you eliminate many of these foods, you may experience withdrawal symptoms such as headaches and fatigue. It's tough, but have faith that this will only last a short time as your body adjusts to whole, nutrient-dense, genetically optimal foods. Most people who report discomfort transitioning over to caveman-style eating say the withdrawal symptoms last anywhere from a couple of days to a few weeks. To help mitigate the withdrawals, increase your vegetable intake to boost your micronutrient levels, and increase your consumption of healthy fats to keep your energy levels balanced. Cravings are also a very common experience, and so we put together a few tips to manage these.

❋ EAT AN EGG
Set a rule for yourself that when you have a craving, satisfy it by eating an egg. After savoring one the most nutritious foods on the planet, chances are you won't want anything else.

❋ HAVE A SERVING OF HEALTHY FATS
We often advise clients to add a spoonful of coconut oil to a cup of green tea or black coffee to curb sugar cravings.

❋ DISTRACT YOURSELF
It's an age-old tip, but it definitely works. Go for a walk, call a friend, have a bath and, before you know it, the craving will pass.

❋ CHOCOLATE TREAT
Try having some coconut oil mixed with a touch of organic cocoa powder. The fat of the oil and the sweetness of the cocoa should help satisfy the craving.

❋ REMEMBER YOUR GOALS
Remind yourself why you set out to do this and how you want to look and feel. If the food you crave is going to hinder your progress, don't eat it!

CHAPTER 8

The Paleo Shopping List

" I never thought I'd hear myself say this but I can't get enough of liver, bacon, and onions—delicious! Don't even get me started on how amazing homemade burgers are, especially after a workout! **KATRINA JASTSENKOVA** (Client) *"*

It's almost time to get started with the amazing recipes we have lined up for you, but before we do, let's go over the grocery list essentials. Be sure to check out the resources located in the back of this book (pages 196-197) to learn where you can source many of these ingredients in your area or online.

GRASS-FED MEAT AND FREE-RANGE POULTRY

All types of unprocessed meat, poultry, and eggs are good for you. By this we are referring to meat in its natural form, not hot dogs, luncheon meats, or chicken nuggets. Place a priority on improving the quality of your ingredients, and buy from farmers markets, butchers, local delicatessens, and independent local grocery stores. We recommend developing a relationship with your local butcher. Ours not only explains how the meat and poultry is sourced, but he also always offers us some great cooking tips and ideas.

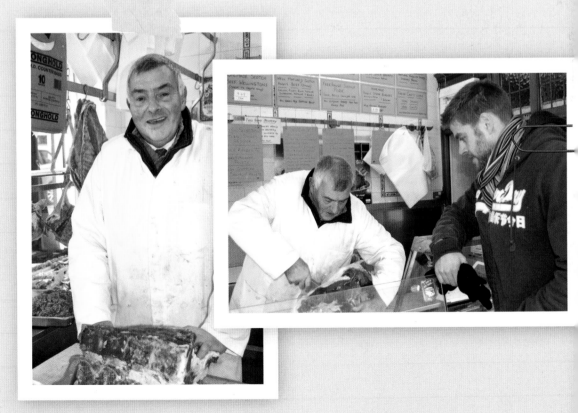

Red meat and poultry are the key sources of essential amino acids in our diet. They also provide a load of vitamins and such minerals as iron, zinc, and selenium.[28] Ideally, your meat should be grass fed and reared outdoors. Grass-fed meats have higher levels of a healthy fat known as conjugated linoleic acid (CLA), which is renowned for its fat-burning properties. They also have higher levels of cancer-fighting antioxidants compared to grain-fed meats. Most importantly, grass-fed meats have a healthier omega-3 to omega-6 ratio.[29] Remember, a crucial factor in weight loss and in achieving optimal health is balancing omega-3 and omega-6 fats across our diet.

Of course, most people find supermarkets to be the most convenient option for buying food, but before you grab another steak or pack of sausages on your way home, understand that most supermarket meat comes from grain-fed animals administered with hormones and antibiotics. You in turn ingest these objectionable additions that disrupt your own hormones and increase the toxic load in your body. If you are shopping at a supermarket, the best option is to look for and buy organic, free-range brands.

Meat, poultry, and eggs are always best purchased from farms where you can ensure the animals were raised without hormones and antibiotics and allowed to routinely spend their days roaming the pasture freely. It's worth noting that the definition of "free range" that your supermarket and government uses is far looser than you might imagine. Technically, even animals raised in crowded, indoor feeding operations can be labeled as "free range" as long as they are given "the ability to access" the outdoors; there is no requirement to how easy that access should be for the animal, how much exposure time it must have each day, or how large the outdoor space must be. In some instances, it may be a sad patch of gravel. Seeking out higher quality meat may mean a little extra effort initially, but the nutritional difference it makes is substantial. And when you support farms that rear their animals in a natural environment with the diet nature intended, you support animal welfare.

EGGS

An egg is a true multivitamin in a shell and a great daily investment in your health. Almost all the nutrients are in the yolk (not the white), so contrary to popular belief, the yolk is the part we definitely should be eating. Cholesterol expert Chris Masterjohn explains the nutritional values of egg yolks in his detailed 2005 article, "The Incredible, Edible Egg."[30] We strongly suggest checking it out, but in a nutshell (or should we say eggshell?), the yolk contains 100 percent of our daily requirement for essential fatty acids, carotenoids, and vitamins A, D, E, and K. It also contains 90 percent of the calcium, iron, phosphorus, zinc, thiamin, B6, folate, and B12, and 89 percent of the pantothenic acid of our daily recommended intake. Hopefully you have stopped worrying about cholesterol by now, but it may also interest you to know that a recent study in *Clinical Nutrition & Metabolic Care* revealed that an increase in consumption of egg yolks had no impact on the cholesterol levels of 70 percent of the population.[31] So let's put an end to these egg-white omelets and start enjoying the tastiest part of the egg again. Forget apples for a moment; one study asserts that three eggs a day can help keep the doctor away.[32]

- - - - - - - - - - - - - - - -

[28] H. Biesalski, "Meat as a component of a healthy diet—are there any risks or benefits if meat is avoided?" *Meat Science* 70.3 (2005): 509-24.
[29] C. Daley, A. Abbott, P. Doyle, G. Nader, S. Larson. "A review of fatty acid profiles and antioxidant content in grass-fed and grain-fed beef." *Nutrition Journal* 9.10 (2010): http://www.nutritionj.com/content/9/1/10
[30] C Masterjohn. "The Incredible, Edible Egg." www.cholesterol-and-health.com (July 2005): http://www.cholesterol-and-health.com/Egg_Yolk.html.
[31] M. Fernandez. "Dietary cholesterol provided by eggs and plasma lipoproteins in healthy populations." *Clinical Nutrition & Metabolic Care* 9.1 (2006) 8-12.
[32] K. Herron, I. Lofgren, M. Sharman, J. Volek, M. Fernandez. "High intake of cholesterol results in less atherogenic low-density lipoprotein particles in men and women independent of response classification." *Metabolism* 53.6 (2004): 823-30.

FISH AND SEAFOOD

Fish is fantastically healthy and clients often feel much better after increasing the amount of fish they eat. Aim to consume at least three portions of oily fish a week, as these are a rich source of omega-3 fats. When trying to remember which fish are highest in omega-3s, remember S.M.A.S.H.

Salmon Mackerel Anchovies Sardines Herring

Ideally, the fish you buy should be fresh and wild-caught. Problem is, most fish available today is farmed, and consequently often kept in overcrowded conditions rife with contaminants. Farm-raised fish are fed antibiotics and other drugs, and then, when they go to market, they get treated with coloring agents.

Another important consideration when purchasing fish and seafood is sustainability. Unethical fishing practices now threaten the future of many species of fish, so we want to do our part by purchasing from responsible sources. To learn more about this, we recommend chef Hugh Fearnley-Whittingstall's excellent guide "Fish to Eat, Fish to Avoid." [33]

The best option is to find good, independent fishmongers or an online supplier like WildPacificSalmon.com, where you can ask questions about how the fish were caught. If purchasing from a supermarket, always check labels—look for line-caught or pole-caught fish, and also hand-dived or creel-caught seafood. If you buy farmed fish, check that the fish has a Marine Stewardship Council (MSC) logo to certify that it was sourced from a sustainable fishery.

Bream, sole, cockles, mackerel, red mullet, mussels, crab, pollock, sardines, herring, and anchovies are among the best supermarket choices. If you are struggling to source wild fish or are limited by a budget, then canned fish is another option since it is usually wild caught. Again, choose a responsible brand.

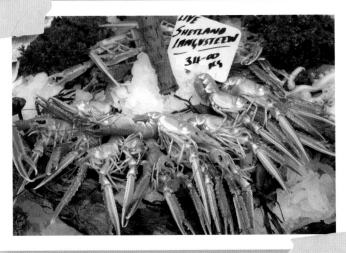
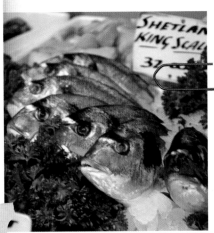

[33] You can download a mobile app or PDF guide at www.fishfight.net/hughs-fish-fight-app

FATS AND OILS

As we have learned, not all fats and oils are created equally. Some are exceptionally beneficial in any form they take. Some are great for dressing a salad but not for cooking. Some make great snacks. And others should be limited or completely avoided. So what to put in your grocery cart? Let's explore!

FATS TO COOK WITH

Monosaturated and polyunsaturated fats, like the vegetable oils that we often cook with, are in fact the worst fats to be used for cooking. When heated they change structure, a process known as oxidation, and this makes them highly inflammatory to the body. On the other hand, cooking with saturated fats (as our grandparents did) is much better as these remain more stable at higher temperatures.

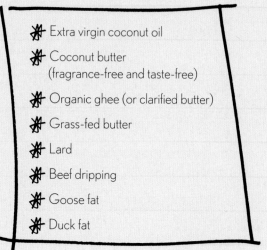

- Extra virgin coconut oil
- Coconut butter (fragrance-free and taste-free)
- Organic ghee (or clarified butter)
- Grass-fed butter
- Lard
- Beef dripping
- Goose fat
- Duck fat

FATS TO EAT

In addition to using fats for cooking or as a dressing, foods high in fat can be included in meals or eaten as a snack, including ...

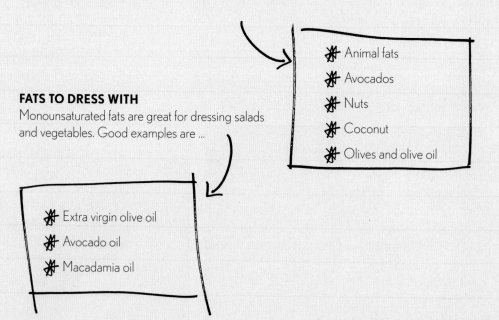

- Animal fats
- Avocados
- Nuts
- Coconut
- Olives and olive oil

FATS TO DRESS WITH

Monounsaturated fats are great for dressing salads and vegetables. Good examples are ...

- Extra virgin olive oil
- Avocado oil
- Macadamia oil

These beneficial oils are best added to a meal after cooking. Similar to polyunsaturated fats, heating these fats can alter their chemical structure and destroy their antioxidant content. To ensure that these oils are protected from light and heat exposure, always buy them in dark bottles and store in the refrigerator.

FATS TO SERIOUSLY LIMIT

In order to improve our ratio of omega-3 to omega-6 fats, we need to limit our intake of omega-6 fats as these are already overly abundant in our diet. Polyunsaturated fats are difficult to avoid entirely, especially if you eat out, so limit their intake whenever possible.

FATS TO AVOID

Avoid all hydrogenated or partially hydrogenated fats and oils. These are usually found in ...

* Seed and vegetable oils–that's corn, sunflower, safflower, soy, and canola **Avoid adding these oils to your shopping cart altogether. Limit foods that contain them as an ingredient**

* Nuts and nut oils (consume in moderation)

* Grain-fed meat

* Factory-farmed poultry and eggs

* Preserved foods (sunflower oil is often used as a preservative, so check labels)

* Store-bought condiments like mayonnaise and salad dressings

* Baked goods like cookies, cakes, pastries, and savory snacks

* Processed foods like breakfast cereals, chips, and other potato products

* Low-fat spreads

* Fast foods and frozen meal products

Hydrogenated fats are chemically processed fats that cause excessive damage to the cells in our bodies. When ingested, they cause an immediate disturbance in healthy cardiovascular function. Long-term consumption is directly associated with obesity, chronic diseases, cancer, and accelerated aging.

DAIRY

If you include dairy in your diet, full-fat organic dairy is the best option. Cream, natural yogurt, and butter offer the most nutritional benefits. Fermented dairy products are excellent for replenishing good bacteria in the gut. They also contain very little lactose as the bacteria consume the lactose during the fermentation process. Kefir (fermented milk) is usually the most widely available. Unpasteurized or raw dairy, although more difficult to obtain, has recently become popular for its health properties. Unlike pasteurized milk, raw milk still contains the lactase enzymes so the body can easily break down the lactose. Research suggests that raw milk may protect the body against viruses and bacteria, providing anti-cancer and antimicrobial properties.[34]

OUR TOP 5 DAIRY CHOICES

* Organic or untreated raw heavy cream
* Grass-fed butter or ghee
* Greek yogurt with live and active cultures
* Kefir with live and active cultures
* Raw milk (unpasteurized)

[34] E. Mattick and J. Golding. "Relative value of raw and heated milk in nutrition." *Lancet 2* (1936) 703-6.

NUTS: "NATURE'S CONDIMENT"

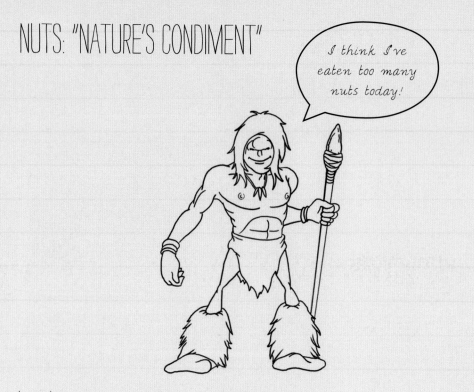

I think I've eaten too many nuts today!

In moderation, nuts can provide a source of minerals and essential fats. Yet we hear the statement above from our clients over and over again. When people switch to eating caveman-style, nuts provide a healthy, convenient snack solution, but they can also be very "moreish," as in the more you eat, the more you want. Although they contain essential minerals such as magnesium and zinc, eating too many can lead to digestive problems. Most nuts contain high levels of omega-6, which we need to limit.

In the *Paleo Primer* recipe collection, nuts are kept to a minimum; they are usually included as a condiment sprinkled over vegetables or on a salad to add flavor. Nut flours like ground almonds are also used occasionally to make a crispy breadcrumb-like topping for fish or chicken or to provide a gluten-free alternative to wheat flour for cakes and cookies.

Some nuts have a slightly better profile of nutrients. Our top three nuts are:

✳ MACADAMIAS
They are high in monounsaturated fats and contain very few omega-6 fats. They are also delicious dipped in dark chocolate.

✳ CHESTNUTS
Compared to other nuts, chestnuts are unique because they consist of more starch than fat, and so make a fantastic source of natural carbohydrates. We like chestnut flour for baking.

✳ BRAZIL NUTS
Brazil nuts are high in a mineral known as selenium, which is important for memory and thyroid health. You only need one or two Brazil nuts to secure your daily requirements for selenium, and their high omega-6 content warrants moderation anyway.

VEGETABLES

Your plate needs plenty of fresh, minimally processed, high-quality vegetables! Ideally, you should source these fresh and locally from farmers markets rather than from supermarkets. Many supermarket vegetables are now imported, traveling long distances from farm to table, so the nutrient content is lower due to premature picking and artificial ripening with ethylene gas. For that reason, even non-organic produce grown locally trumps imported produce. Also avoid buying precut and bagged vegetables that have been chopped and peeled as this exposes them to air that degrades vitamins and minerals. If convenience is important to you, we recommend frozen organic veggies, which are typically picked at the peak of the season and flash frozen to lock in nutrients.

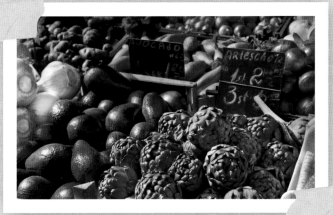

FRUIT

Although fruit is a source of antioxidants, vitamins, and minerals, liberal consumption of it can result in excessive carb intake and hampered weight loss efforts. Remember, our ancestors ate wild fruit, far less sweet than today's cultivated crops. And because they did not have year-round access to fruits, they only ate them during narrow ripening seasons. Fructose, the carbohydrate source in fruit, causes digestive issues for many people and has been shown to increase appetite. As most of our clients ask us to help them kick their sweet tooths, we find that cutting down on fruit can really help. You can get all the same nutrients from vegetables, without the sugar, so we like to keep fruit on the "occasional" list, mainly using it in our dessert recipes for special occasions.

There are a few exceptions: lemons, limes, avocados, and seasonal berries are all very low in sugar and packed with other antioxidants, so these are good to include on a regular basis.

EAT FRUIT, DON'T DRINK IT
Fruit juice (even fresh squeezed) is nothing but a large serving of sugar quickly released into the bloodstream. Many fruit juices and smoothies are also pasteurized to increase their shelf life, and this destroys most of the vitamin content, especially vitamin C. Remember, it's better to consume food as nature intended, that is, whole pieces of fruit with all the digestive enzymes and fiber intact.

FARTY FRUIT AND VEGETABLES (FODMAPS)

Some vegetables contain compounds that many of us find difficult to digest. These are referred to as FODMAPs, or fermentable oligosaccharides, disaccharides, monosaccharides, and polyols—try saying that one quickly! Each of these is a type of carbohydrate that is not easily absorbed by the bowel. The bacteria in your bowels then ferment these carbohydrates, creating wind and bloating.

If you struggle with abdominal distension and bloating after eating foods containing FODMAPs, you might need to limit or avoid these foods completely. Such discomfort is usually a sign you have an overgrowth of bad bacteria and need to adapt your nutrition even further. Sébastien Noël, author of *The Paleo Recipe Book*, provides a fantastic guide to resolving this problem in his blog article entitled "You and Your Gut Flora."[35] Generally, we each have an individual tolerance for FODMAP carbohydrates, so if you are experiencing digestive issues, it is worthwhile to eliminate the foods below for a few weeks and then slowly reintroduce them in small amounts while monitoring your symptoms.

Fruit

- Most fruit juice
- Dried fruits
- Apples (also apple juice and sauce)
- Apricots
- Cherries
- Dates
- Grapes
- Lychee
- Mango
- Peaches
- Pears
- Plums
- Prunes
- Watermelon

Vegetables

- Artichokes
- Asparagus
- Beetroot
- Broccoli
- Brussels sprouts
- Cabbage
- Cauliflower
- Fennel
- Garlic
- Sugar snap peas
- Leeks
- Okra
- Onions
- Peas
- Shallots

Other FODMAP Foods

- Honey
- Foods flavored with fructose or sorbitol
- Sweeteners such as sorbitol, mannitol, xylitol, maltitol, and isomalt (used in sugar-free chewing gum, sweets, and mints)

[35] www.paleodietlifestyle.com/you-and-your-gut-flora

THE ORGANIC QUESTION

We all know there's a higher price tag on organics, so it's sometimes a good idea to prioritize. Helpfully, the Environmental Working Group (EWG), a US-based nonprofit organization, tests the pesticide residue of conventionally grown produce every year and publishes its findings. Below are the current recommendations for 2013.[36] The Dirty Dozen-Plus features items that should be purchased organic due to their high pesticide load. The Clean Fifteen, however, contains the safest non-organic choices, testing for little or no traces of pesticide. Most of the Clean Fifteen fall into this category because they have a tough, inedible exterior that protects the edible portion from pesticide exposure.

The Clean Fifteen

- Asparagus
- Avocados
- Cabbage
- Cantaloupe
- Sweet corn
- Eggplant
- Grapefruit
- Kiwi
- Mangos
- Mushrooms
- Onions
- Papayas
- Pineapples
- Sweet peas (frozen)
- Sweet potatoes

The Dirty Dozen

- Apples
- Celery
- Cherry tomatoes
- Cucumbers
- Grapes
- Hot peppers
- Nectarines
- Peaches
- Potatoes
- Spinach
- Strawberries
- Sweet bell peppers

plus

- Summer squash
- Kale/Greens

---

36 www.ewg.org/foodnews/summary.php

THE PALEO SPICE RACK

You should always have herbs and spices stocked up at home. They transform the flavor of food and provide an excellent source of nutritional antioxidants. Many herbs have medicinal properties, providing an anti-inflammatory or antiviral effect in the body and protecting against disease. The cheaper, more sustainable option is to grow your own herbs (or even just replant any potted herbs you buy). If this isn't viable, opt for dried herbs.

To save some preparation time on days you're against the clock, you can buy dried garlic granules and ginger powder, but always keep in mind that fresh herbs, spices, garlic, and ginger will always bring the most benefits. Always have the following dried herbs and spices on hand. Also, remember to replace every six months, as over time spices can sustain oxidative damage. Try to purchase organic spices, which have higher micronutrient values by virtue of not being irradiated like most conventional spices.

- Chinese five spice
- Cayenne pepper
- Nutmeg
- Smoked paprika
- Cumin
- Mustard powder
- Celtic sea salt or Himalayan pink salt

- Thyme
- Basil
- Cinnamon
- Mustard seeds
- Turmeric
- Curry powder
- Mixed herbs (also Italian blends)

- Paprika
- Allspice
- Chilli powder
- Parsley
- Black pepper
- Oregano
- Rosemary

Aim to grow or buy these items fresh and frequently:

- Garlic
- Ginger
- Onions
- Herbs when possible (parsley, rosemary, thyme, tarragon, mint, cilantro, basil)

TIPS ON SALT

You'll notice that we suggest seasoning with unprocessed salt in some of our recipes. The amount you use is very much up to your individual taste. The reasoning here is that when you eliminate processed foods from your diet you will naturally lower your salt intake, reduce systemic inflammation, and lower water and sodium retention. Furthermore, if you regularly perform high-intensity exercise, you may need additional dietary sodium to replenish the sodium lost through perspiration. Adding a little good, high-quality salt to your meals will help maintain your body's sodium requirements.

The type of salts we recommend are unprocessed and natural salts such as Celtic sea salt, Himalayan pink salt, or vegetable salts like Herbamere (widely available in health food stores). All of these have a slightly higher mineral content. Avoid common table salt as this is highly processed and often contains additives.

TEN REASONS TO HERB AND SPICE UP YOUR LIFE

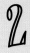 **1 DON'T WORRY, BE HAPPY WITH CILANTRO**
Coriander boosts our production of the "good mood" chemical serotonin in the brain.

2 CURB CRAVINGS WITH CINNAMON
Cinnamon is one of the highest antioxidant spices and improves insulin sensitivity. By increasing the body's metabolic efficiency, it lowers levels of sugar in the blood.

 3 DETOX WITH PARSLEY
Parsley is a powerful diuretic herb. It decreases water retention by supporting detoxification processes in the kidneys.

 4 NO MORE NAUSEA WITH CUMIN
Cumin is superb for digestion and used in ancient traditions to treat stomach pain, indigestion, diarrhea, nausea, and morning sickness.

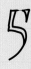 **5 JUST TOTALLY AWESOME TUMERIC**
Turmeric is the anti-inflammatory powerhouse! Research has repeatedly shown that the curcumin ingredient in turmeric is effective in both preventing and decreasing the growth of cancer.

 6 GARLIC FOR COLDS AND FLU
Garlic is your best friend when it comes to fighting colds or flu. It has an antimicrobial effect against bacteria and viruses. To make the most of garlic's disease-defending properties, it should be crushed or chopped and left to stand for a few minutes before cooking.

7 PAINKILLER GINGER
Ginger is a potent anti-inflammatory agent. A large chunk steeped in hot water is a great way to soothe inflammatory conditions such as arthritis, throat infections, or joint pains.

 8 MUSTARD MEDICINE
Mustard seeds have long been considered more of a medicinal plant than a food. Similar to other brassica vegetables (cabbage, broccoli, and kale), it contains many cancer-fighting compounds and is also considered an aphrodisiac in Chinese medicine.

 9 ROSEMEMORY
Rosemary supports healthy brain function by preventing the breakdown of neurotransmitters in the brain. This helps to boost memory and protect against dementia.

10 GOOD OLD SAGE
Sage is known as a purifying herb due to its detoxifying effect on the body. It has been used to treat conditions like gingivitis (gum disease) and rheumatoid arthritis.

PALEO FOODS TO ADD TO YOUR SHOPPING CART

Protein

EGGS
- Duck
- Chicken
- Goose

POULTRY
- Chicken
- Duck
- Turkey

MEAT/GAME
- Lamb
- Beef
- Pork
- Buffalo
- Venison
- Pheasant
- Grouse
- Organ meats (liver and kidney)
- Veal
- Gluten-free sausages (more than 80% meat)
- Unsmoked bacon

FISH/SEAFOOD
- Anchovies
- Salmon
- Sardines
- Mackerel
- Herring
- Shrimp
- Sea bass
- Scallops
- Mussels
- Cockles
- Crab
- Squid
- Cod
- Pollock
- Haddock
- Lemon sole
- Dover sole
- Halibut
- Trout
- Tuna

Fats

OILS
- Extra virgin olive oil
- Extra virgin coconut oil
- Avocado oil
- Macadamia oil

SOLID FATS
- Ghee
- Grass-fed butter (Kerrygold)
- Coconut manna

OTHER
- Grass-fed heavy cream
- Coconut milk
- Coconut flakes
- Coconut cream (tin or carton)
- Coconut cream (bar)
- Desiccated coconut

NUTS/NUT BUTTERS
- Almonds
- Brazil nuts
- Cashews
- Chestnuts
- Hazelnuts
- Macadamias
- Pecans
- Pistachios
- Walnuts

Carbohydrates

VEGETABLES
- Artichoke
- Arugala
- Asparagus
- Broccoli
- Brussels sprouts
- Butternut squash
- Cabbage
- Carrots
- Cauliflower
- Celery
- Celeriac
- Cucumber
- Eggplant
- Kale
- Lettuce
- Mushrooms
- Red onions
- White onions
- Parsnips
- Peppers
- Radish
- Spinach
- Sweet potato
- Swiss chard
- Watercress
- Zucchini

FRUITS
- Lemons
- Limes
- Avocados
- Blackberries
- Blueberries
- Raspberries
- Strawberries
- Tomatoes
- Gooseberries

ALL OTHER FRUITS OCCASIONALLY

PART 1 CONCLUSION & TAKEAWAYS

There you have it. We have guided you through everything you need to know to get you started on your new Primal/paleo journey. Now for the really exciting bit ... the food! Before we move on, we just wanted to put all the information in a nutshell for you.

- Avoid processed foods like luncheon meats, bread, cookies, chips, soft drinks, and sweets.
- Avoid hydrogenated fats
- Avoid artificial sweeteners
- Avoid sugar as much as possible
- Avoid gluten-containing grains
- Avoid low-fat and homogenized dairy
- Avoid vegetable oils, seed oils, and other foods high in omega-6 fats
- Eat quality grass-fed meat and free-range poultry
- Eat omega-3-rich fish (SMASH) two or three times a week
- Eat plenty of vegetables
- Eat grass-fed, full-fat dairy such as butter and heavy cream
- Carbohydrates are not the enemy—just don't eat more than you need, and make sure they are from safe sources such as sweet potato, vegetables, and rice
- Saturated fats are your friend
- Monounsaturated fats are also your friend
- Eat plenty of herbs and spices
- Limit your fruit intake. Stick to lemons, limes, avocados, and seasonal berries—all other fruit only occasionally
- Moderation is the key. (Something to keep in mind when you get to our dessert section)
- Plan, prepare, and cook. Planning your meals and cooking extra for lunches and snacks or to freeze will always keep you ahead of the game

TIME TO JUMP IN

Almost every recipe you are about to see was written, cooked, and photographed by the two of us. We loved the journey we've taken in creating this book, and we are certain it will serve you well. It works for us and for many of our clients—now it's your turn.

BREAKFASTS

HOW TO POACH AN EGG

Poaching allows you to obtain the most nutritional value from an egg (unless, of course, you are up for consuming them raw, Rocky Balboa-style). And lucky for you, there's more than one way to poach an egg.

OPTION 1: THE PROPER POACHED EGG

YOU WILL NEED
A saucepan
1 tablespoon apple cider vinegar
Eggs

1 Fill the saucepan with water and add the apple cider vinegar. Heat until the water begins to simmer.

2 Stir the water so a whirlpool starts to form, and crack the egg into the middle. The water movement will cause the egg to wrap into a ball.

3 Leave the egg poaching in the water until the white has cooked fully. This usually takes around 2-3 minutes; however, we like our yolks runny, so leave it in slightly longer if you prefer a more solid yolk.

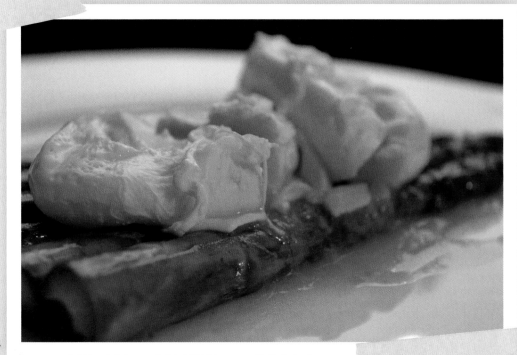

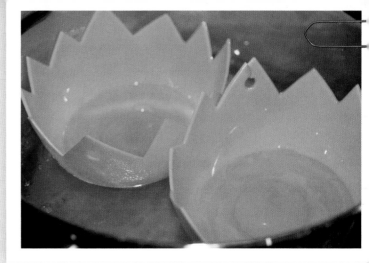

OPTION 2: SILICONE EGG POACHERS

YOU WILL NEED
Silicone egg poachers
Saucepan with a lid
Macadamia or olive oil
Eggs

1 Fill the saucepan with water and heat until the water begins to simmer.

2 Coat the silicone egg poacher with a small amount of oil to prevent the egg from sticking. Crack open an egg and pour into the silicone poacher.

3 Place the poachers in the saucepan of water and cover.

4 Leave poaching in the water until the white has cooked fully. This usually takes around 3-5 minutes; leave in slightly longer if you prefer a more solid yolk.

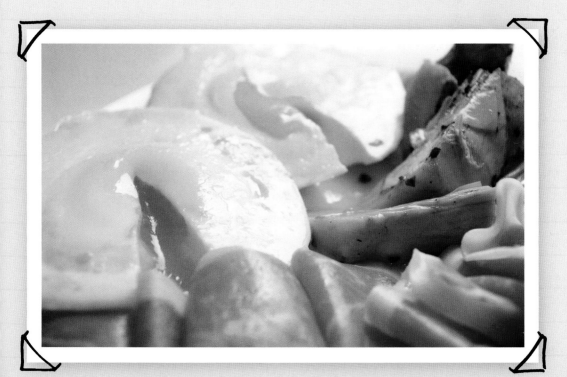

PARSLEY SALMON AND POACHED EGGS

This is one of the healthiest breakfasts you can eat, not to mention incredibly quick to put together. And it will easily keep you fueled until lunchtime. You'll need a steamer for this one.

1 5-ounce salmon fillet
1 teaspoon dried parsley
2 large handfuls of spinach
2 eggs
1 tablespoon apple cider vinegar
Salt and pepper to taste

1 Bring water in a steamer to a simmer. Cover the salmon in parsley and place in the steamer. Leave some room to add the spinach later.

2 While the salmon is cooking, poach the eggs (see How to Poach an Egg, page 64).

3 While the eggs are poaching, add spinach to the steamer.

4 When the eggs are cooked, place them on a plate; add the cooked salmon and spinach.

PREPARATION TIME: 2 minutes
COOKING TIME: 10 minutes
SERVES: 1 (or double up and take a portion for lunch)

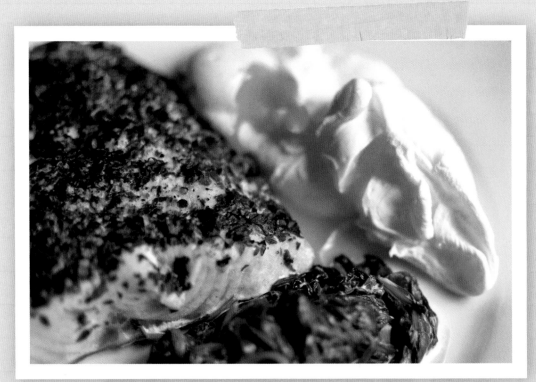

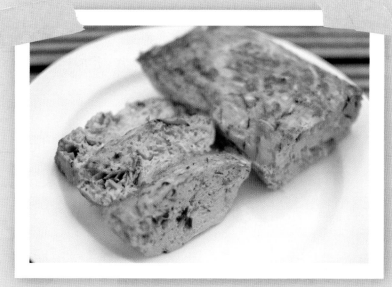

OMEGA BREAKFAST BAKE

We bake a large serving of this omega-3-boosting meal in a loaf pan so it can be served in slices. Make this at the beginning of the week, and you can keep the loaf in the fridge. It's ideal as an instant breakfast or a convenient snack when you come home from work.

Coconut oil or butter to grease the
  loaf pan
8 eggs
Salt and pepper to taste
1 zucchini, grated (with skin on)
2 5-ounce mackerel fillets, cooked
  (Feel free to use fresh, cured, or
  canned. You can also substitute with
  salmon, sardines, herring, or any other
  cooked meat.)

PREPARATION TIME: 10 minutes
COOKING TIME: 30 minutes
SERVES: 4

1 Preheat oven to 350°F.

2 Grease a loaf pan with butter or coconut oil.

3 Place the eggs in a large mixing bowl, and mix until the whites and yolks are blended.

4 Season with a sprinkle of salt and pepper.

5 Add the grated zucchini to the beaten egg.

6 Break the mackerel into pieces, and stir into the egg and zucchini mixture.

7 Pour into prepared loaf pan, and bake for around 20-30 minutes.

8 Use a knife to check that it is cooked in the middle; the knife should come out clean.

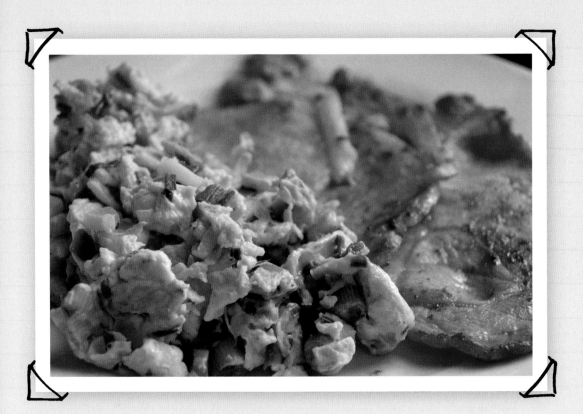

Quick-Cook Chive Scrambled Eggs and Bacon

Here's a simple yet hearty breakfast that can be cooked in minutes and leave you happy for hours. This recipe uses chives and scallions, both from the onion family. The difference is, chives are milder and more slender than scallions.

Coconut oil for the pan
2 slices of unsmoked bacon
3 eggs
Handful of fresh chives, chopped
2 scallions, chopped
Salt and pepper to taste

PREPARATION TIME: 3 minutes
COOKING TIME: 5 minutes
SERVES: 1

1 Place the coconut oil in a pan and melt over low heat, then add the bacon.

2 As your bacon cooks, beat three eggs in a bowl and add the chives and scallions.

3 When the bacon is cooked to your liking, remove from the pan and add the egg and scallion-chive mixture. Keep stirring in the pan until it's scrambled.

4 Season with a little salt and pepper, and serve with the cooked bacon.

Creamy Green Omelet

This is a bit of a twist on an old favorite. Adding grated creamed coconut and cilantro give this dish a distinctive twist. Sometimes we add some steamed whitefish or chicken and enjoy this as a quick supper.

Coconut oil for the pan
Handful of spinach
3 eggs
1 tablespoon creamed coconut, grated
¼ cup chopped fresh cilantro
2 ounces cooked fish or chicken
   (optional)

1 Melt the coconut oil in pan over low heat.

2 Add the spinach and cook until the leaves wilt down.

3 While the spinach is cooking, beat the eggs in a bowl and then stir in the grated creamed coconut and fresh cilantro.

4 Pour the egg mixture over the wilted spinach.

5 Allow the eggs to cook through slowly for around 5 minutes, using a spatula to gently peel them away from the edge of the pan to ensure that they don't stick.

6 Fold in half and serve.

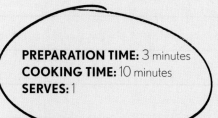

PREPARATION TIME: 3 minutes
COOKING TIME: 10 minutes
SERVES: 1

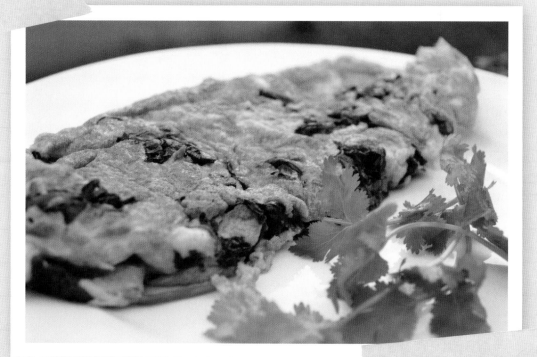

Breakfast Calzone

Pizza for breakfast—
enough said!

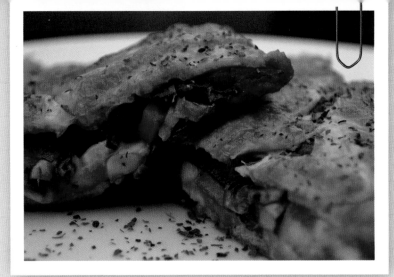

Coconut oil for the pan
4 eggs
2 heaping tablespoons Tomato Sauce
   (page 175 or store-bought)
Large handful of spinach
3-4 thin slices goat cheese (optional)
Small handful of fresh basil
   (or 1 teaspoon dried mixed herbs)
½ red pepper, chopped
5 green olives, halved

- - - - - - - - -

PREPARATION TIME: 2 minutes
COOKING TIME: 8-10 minutes
SERVES: 1-2

- - - - - - - - -

OTHER TASTY FILLINGS IDEAS
* Tuna, feta, and red onion
* Grilled sausage and sweet potato
* Bacon and mushroom
* Leftover Italian Meatballs
   (page 122)
* Avocado, tomato, and mozzarella

1 Melt about a teaspoon of coconut oil in a pan.

2 Beat the eggs in a large bowl until the whites and yolks are combined. Pour the mixture into the pan.

3 Allow to cook through for a few minutes until the egg has set (slightly runny on top). Use a spatula to gently peel the eggs away from the edge of the pan to ensure they don't stick.

4 Spread the tomato sauce over the omelet base as if it were a pizza.

5 Tear up the spinach leaves. Sprinkle the torn spinach, goat cheese, and fresh basil (or mixed herbs) onto the cooked omelet. Add the pepper and olives, and gently fold the omelet in half, sealing the edges by pressing down with the spatula.

6 Allow to cook for another 5 minutes to ensure that the cheese has melted.

7 Best served hot from the pan, but like pizza it's just as tasty served cold.

WARNING
Eat this alone, because you'll be unable to contain yourself!

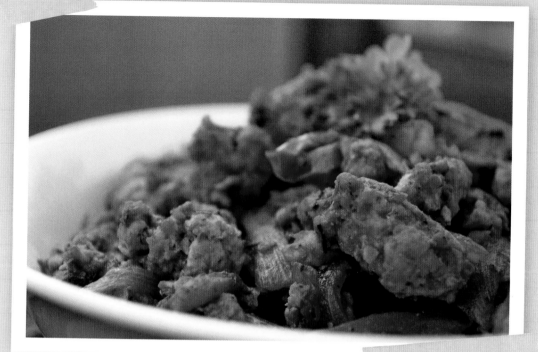

BREAKFAST STIR-FRY

A tasty egg-free breakfast that can be thrown into a pan and cooked in minutes. Ideal as a hearty start to your day.

Coconut oil for the pan
½ red or white onion, peeled and chopped
2 tomatoes, chopped
½ pound ground chicken or turkey
3 tablespoons Tomato Sauce (page 175 or store-bought)
1 teaspoon mixed herbs
Salt and pepper to taste

1 Heat a little coconut oil in a frying pan.

2 Add the onion and tomato to the pan and stir-fry.

3 Add the ground chicken or turkey, and continue to stir-fry for 2-3 minutes.

4 Add the tomato sauce, mixed herbs, salt, and pepper, and stir-fry for another 5 minutes until the meat is cooked through.

PREPARATION TIME: 3 minutes
COOKING TIME: 10 minutes
SERVES: 1-2

 TIP Tastes great with sliced avocado served on top.

BREAKFAST BURGER

Bacon, avocado, and tomato sandwiched between two juicy layers of meat. Never mind hours, this will keep you going for days!

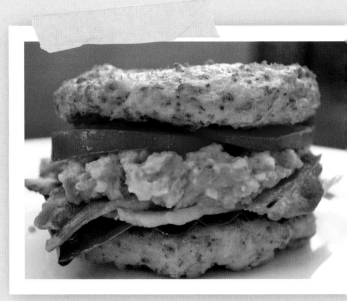

1 pound ground chicken or turkey
2 tablespoons mixed herbs
Salt and pepper to taste
2 ripe avocados
6 slices of bacon
Large handful of spinach
2 large tomatoes, sliced

PREPARATION TIME: 8 minutes
COOKING TIME: 20 minutes
SERVES: 3-4

≪ TIP ≫

Try adding a tablespoon of fresh cilantro, a squeeze of fresh lemon juice, or ½ teaspoon of chili to the avocado mixture for an extra flavor hit.

1 Preheat oven to 350°F.

2 Using your hands, combine the ground chicken or turkey, mixed herbs, salt, and pepper in a bowl.

3 Form the mixture into six to eight circular burger shapes, but flatten them down so they are around 1-inch thick. (These will form the "bun" for the burger.)

4 Place the burgers on a grill tray and bake for about 20 minutes, or you can panfry the patties if you're pushed for time (this takes around 10 minutes).

5 While the burgers are cooking, start to prepare your filling.

6 Scoop all the flesh out of the avocados into a bowl, add salt and pepper, and simply mash it together until creamy (keep it a little chunky, like guacamole).

7 Cook the bacon in a frying pan until nice and golden.

8 Remove the burger "buns" from the oven.

9 Assemble the layers in this order: meat bun, spinach leaves, two slices of bacon, two spoonfuls of mashed avocado, tomato slices, and top with another meat bun.

10 Admire your creation for a few minutes, then wolf it down while it's still hot!

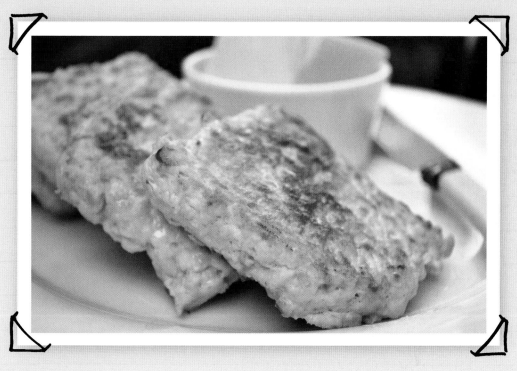

Turkey Toast

Not exactly toast, yet incredibly tasty! The key is to get the seasoning right and serve it hot with some melted butter or ghee.

Oil for the pan (ghee, butter, or goose fat work best)
1 pound ground turkey
1 teaspoon mixed herbs
Salt and pepper to taste

PREPARATION TIME: 4 minutes
COOKING TIME: 6-8 minutes
SERVES: 4

TIP
Try adding other herbs like thyme, rosemary, or parsley to the meat. Mushrooms and sun-dried tomatoes are also great in turkey toast.

1 Heat the oil in a frying pan over a low heat.

2 Combine the meat, herbs, salt, and pepper together in a bowl using your hands.

3 There are two ways to make these into slices of toast. You can flatten the ground turkey mixture onto a sheet of parchment paper and then use a sharp knife to cut into squares. Use a spatula to scoop up each square and place in the pan. Alternatively, you can simply flatten out the ground meat onto a sheet of parchment paper and then place into the pan as one large square, cutting into smaller squares as it cooks in the pan.

4 Cook for around 10 minutes, flipping over each piece after 5 minutes. Ideally they should be golden brown on both sides and cooked through.

5 Once cooked, remove the toast from the pan and spread with butter or ghee. These are best eaten warm from the pan.

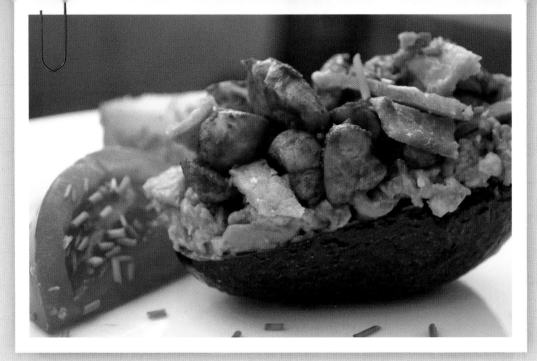

Avocado Breakfast Bowl

Chunky chicken and slices of bacon in a bowl full of healthy fats. Quick, tasty, super filling.

Oil for the pan (ghee,
    butter, or coconut oil)
2 chicken breasts, chopped
Salt and pepper to taste
2 teaspoons smoked paprika
1 ripe avocado
3 slices of bacon, chopped

1 Heat the oil in a frying pan and add the chicken.

2 Stir-fry the chicken and season it with salt, pepper, and smoked paprika.

3 Cook the bacon in a separate frying pan until nice and golden.

4 While the chicken and bacon are cooking, slice the avocado in half and remove the pit. Keeping the skin of the avocado halves intact, scoop out all the flesh into a bowl. Mash together until creamy, keeping it a little chunky.

PREPARATION TIME: 3 minutes
COOKING TIME: 10 minutes
SERVES: 2

5 Place the mashed avocado back into the empty shells. When the chicken and bacon are cooked, place on top of the mashed avocado.

Serve with
Sliced tomato

Crunchy Nut Coconut Flakes

Occasionally you might fancy something a little crunchy for breakfast, so this is our breakfast cereal substitute. It's also great as a quick energy snack.

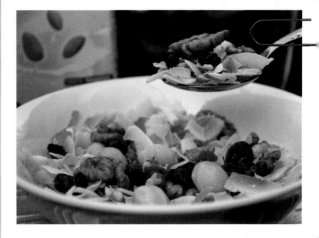

3 tablespoons toasted coconut flakes (toast your own to make it crunchy or buy ready-made)
1 tablespoon walnuts
2 tablespoons whole macadamias
1 teaspoon raisins
1 ounce unsweetened almond milk or Kara coconut milk to serve

Combine all the dry ingredients in a bowl and top with almond or coconut milk. Enjoy!

PREPARATION TIME: 3 minutes
COOKING TIME: N/A
SERVES: 1

Scrambled Eggs with Sun-Dried Tomatoes and Chorizo

A recent brunch discovery at a London café. What a fantastic take on scrambled eggs!

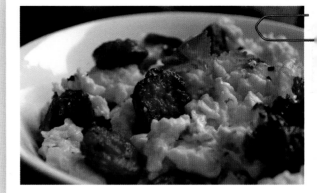

2 chorizo sausages, chopped
Coconut oil for the pan
6 eggs
2-3 Sun-Dried Tomatoes (page 168)

PREPARATION TIME: 3 minutes
COOKING TIME: 5 minutes
SERVES: 1-2

1 Heat a saucepan over medium heat and add the chorizo. Stir occasionally to prevent the meat from overcooking.

2 In a second pan, melt the coconut oil. In a bowl, beat together the eggs and add to the pan. Keep stirring until scrambled.

3 Cut the sun-dried tomatoes into small pieces and stir into the eggs.

4 Serve the eggs topped with the chorizo.

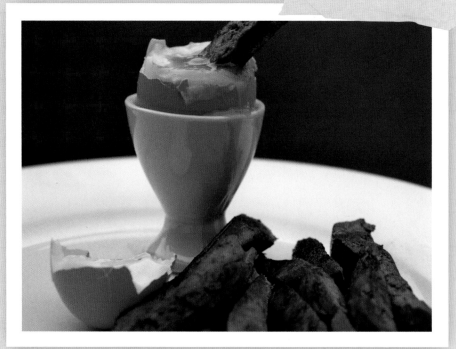

LIVER DIPPY EGG

Liver is not liked by many people, which is a nutritional tragedy as it is packed with vitamins and minerals. It also makes great soldiers that taste great dipped in an egg yolk.

Coconut oil for the pan
7 ounces lamb or beef liver
  (lamb's liver is often cheaper)
2 eggs

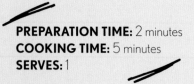

PREPARATION TIME: 2 minutes
COOKING TIME: 5 minutes
SERVES: 1

1 Melt a teaspoon of coconut oil in a pan.

2 Place sliced liver in the pan and gently cook over low heat.

3 Bring a small pot of water to a boil, and place the eggs in the pot.

4 Use an egg timer or boil the eggs for roughly 3 minutes. (Getting the perfect dippy egg isn't easy, so persevere! Not all eggs are the same!)

5 Once the egg is ready, place one in an egg cup, slice off the top, and dunk in a tasty slice of liver.

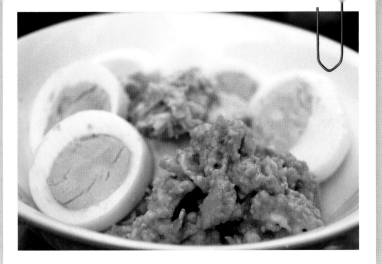

TUNA AVO EGG BRUNCH

This is one of the quick brunches we whip up on weekends when we have a busy day ahead. It offers a good dose of protein and healthy monounsaturated fats will keep you going for hours without even thinking about your next meal.

4 eggs
1 avocado
Juice of 1 lime
1 5-ounce can of tuna packed in water
Pinch of chili powder
 or ½ teaspoon of chili flakes

1 Place the eggs in a pot of boiling water. Boil for 5 minutes and then place in cold water to cool.

2 Slice the avocado in half, remove the pit, and scoop out the flesh into a bowl. Add the lime juice and a pinch of chili, and mash together with a fork.

3 Open the can of tuna and drain off the excess water. Place half of the tuna into each bowl.

4 Slice the boiled eggs and place two in each bowl with 2 tablespoons of the avocado mixture.

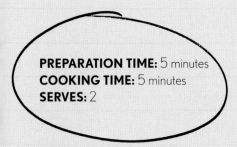

PREPARATION TIME: 5 minutes
COOKING TIME: 5 minutes
SERVES: 2

LIGHT BITES

Citrus Ceviche with Tomato and Avocado Salad

It doesn't get much easier than not cooking at all. This is pure chemistry in action as the citric acid in the lemon and lime juices denature the proteins in the seafood and "cook" the fish without heat. We recommend freezing the fish first to destroy any potential parasites.

2 5-ounce wild-caught salmon fillets, defrosted
Juice of 1 lime
Juice of 1 lemon
½ avocado
¼ cucumber
5 cherry tomatoes
Sliced red onion (optional)
Jalapeños (optional)
Handful of cilantro, chopped
1 tablespoon extra virgin olive oil
Salt and pepper to taste

1 Remove the skin from the salmon, and cut the fillets into 1-inch cubes. Place in a glass dish or freezer bag, and cover with the lemon and lime juice. This will effectively "cook" the salmon, so make sure to cover all the fish.

2 Marinate for at least 6 hours or ideally overnight in the fridge.

3 To make the salad, chop the avocado, cucumber, and cherry tomatoes into small cubes and toss to combine (add onions and jalapeños if desired). When ready to serve, place the salmon on the avocado, tomato, and cucumber. Top with chopped cilantro, a drizzle of olive oil, and salt and pepper to your liking.

PREPARATION TIME: 10 minutes
(marinate overnight or for at least 6 hours)
COOKING TIME: 0 minutes
SERVES: 2

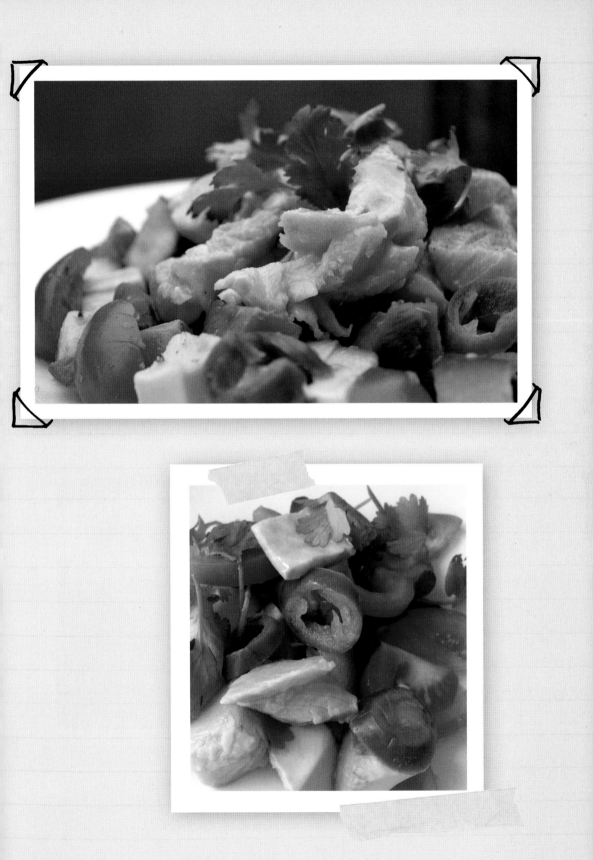

SHRIMP COCKTAIL

A retro classic, no special occasion would be the same without a shrimp cocktail to start. The cocktail sauce is the tricky bit, as some people prefer it spicier than others. Play around with seasoning and tomato paste to tailor your classic cocktail specific to your taste.

For the Cocktail Sauce
2 tablespoons Homemade Mayonnaise (page 173)
1 tablespoon tomato paste
Pinch of cayenne pepper
Tabasco or cayenne pepper to taste

7 ounces cooked shrimp

For the Salad
Lettuce
Juice of half a lemon
½ red bell pepper, chopped
Fresh parsley

1 In a bowl, mix together the Homemade Mayonnaise with tomato paste and cayenne pepper.

2 At this point, you'll customize your own perfect sauce by adding a dash of Tabasco or cayenne pepper, mixing further and tasting. If you prefer a spicy sauce, add more cayenne or Tabasco. If you prefer more of a tomato-based dressing, add more tomato paste.

3 Once you are happy with the sauce, mix in the shrimp and serve over a large salad topped with fresh lemon juice and parsley.

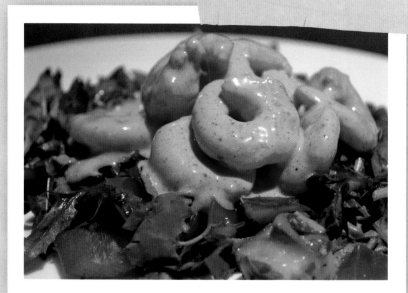

PREPARATION TIME: 5 minutes
COOKING TIME: 0 minutes
SERVES: 2

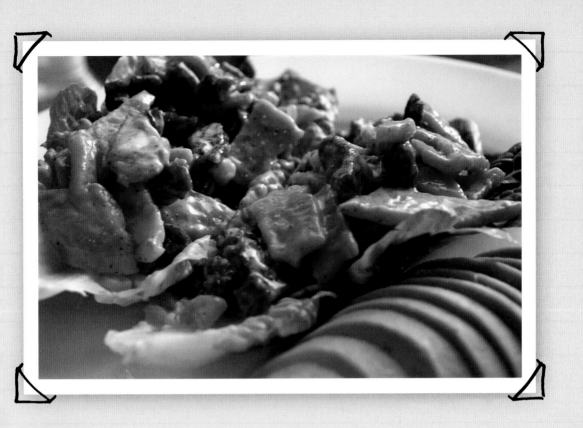

BLT

You can still enjoy your favorite sandwich without eating the bread—simply wrap it with lettuce instead. It's all about the filling, and BLT is always a winner.

6 slices of unsmoked bacon
2 tablespoons Homemade Mayonnaise
 (page 173)
4 Sun-Dried Tomatoes, chopped
 (page 168)

1 Place the bacon in a pan over low heat and cook for 5-8 minutes.

2 Once cooked, cut the bacon into pieces and mix with the mayonnaise and chopped sun-dried tomatoes.

3 Spoon into a lettuce bowl or wrap, top with sliced avocado, and enjoy.

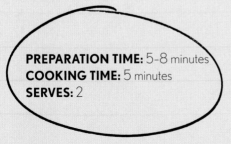

PREPARATION TIME: 5-8 minutes
COOKING TIME: 5 minutes
SERVES: 2

"OMG! WHERE'S THE PROTEIN?" SALAD

Here we focus on adding some fantastic flavors to a bunch of leafy greens.

2 handfuls of mixed greens such as
    watercress, spinach, or arugula
4 ½-inch slices of goat cheese
A few crushed roasted walnuts
2 beetroots, sliced
½ avocado, cubed
1 tablespoon olive oil
1 tablespoon chopped fresh thyme
Salt and pepper to taste

1 Preheat the grill or oven and place the slices of goat cheese in an ovenproof dish. Combine the mixed greens, walnuts, beetroot, and avocado in a bowl.

2 Once the cheese starts to melt and brown, remove from the heat before it gets too soft and loses its round shape. Place on top of the salad.

3 Mix the fresh thyme, olive oil, salt, and pepper together in a bowl, and drizzle over the salad before serving.

PREPARATION TIME: 5 minutes
COOKING TIME: 5 minutes
SERVES: 1

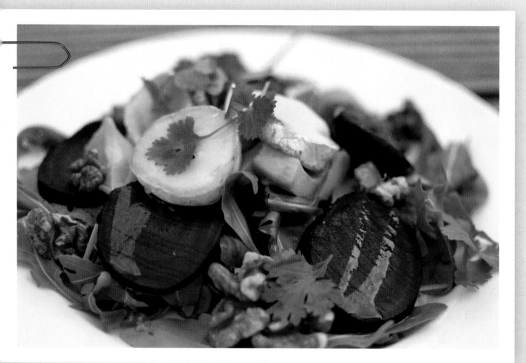

Egg-Stuffed Toms

A classic sandwich filling served without the sandwich! This makes a great appetizer when you're entertaining or a great snack on the go—just place the lid back on the tomato.

2 eggs
2 large beef tomatoes
1 tablespoon Homemade Mayonnaise
   (page 173)
2 teaspoons chopped fresh chives

PREPARATION TIME: 5 minutes
COOKING TIME: 5 minutes
SERVES: 1

1 Place the eggs in a pot of boiling water. Boil for 5 minutes and then place in cold water to cool.

2 While the eggs are boiling, slice the tops off the tomatoes and use a spoon to scoop out the flesh and seeds until you have a hollow shell.

3 Once the eggs have cooled, peel, chop, and mix them with the mayonnaise.

4 Place the mixture inside the tomato, and top with the chopped chives.

5 Use the lid either as a base or place back on the tomato if eating on the go.

6 Top with some chopped fresh parsley and serve.

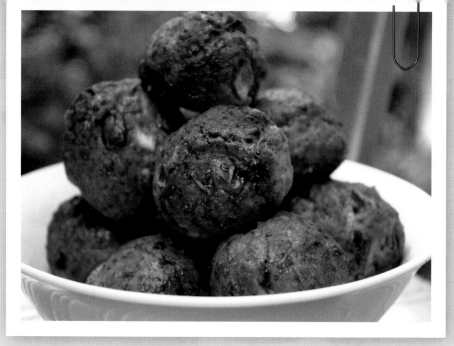

≪ TIP ≫

Celery and
mushrooms are
a nice addition
if you are using
chicken or turkey.
You can also use
dried mixed herbs
if fresh herbs
aren't available.

Crispy Stuffing Balls

Stuffing is so tasty on its own that you don't need to serve it with a Sunday roast. We often make a batch of these at the beginning of the week and keep them in the fridge as a quick, tasty snack. Ground pork is the tastiest, but you can try different combinations of meat with herbs and spices.

1 pound ground pork
1 tablespoon chopped fresh rosemary
1 tablespoon chopped fresh thyme
1 red onion, finely chopped
Salt and pepper to taste
7 ounces peeled, roasted chestnuts

1 Preheat oven to 350°F.

2 Add all the ingredients except for the chestnuts in a bowl, and mix together well using your hands.

3 Chop the chestnuts into small chunks, and mix thoroughly with the other ingredients.

4 Roll the mixture into separate balls, each roughly the size of a golf ball.

5 Place on a baking sheet. Bake for 20-25 minutes until nice and crispy on the outside.

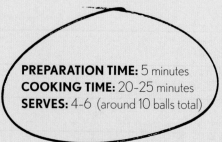

PREPARATION TIME: 5 minutes
COOKING TIME: 20-25 minutes
SERVES: 4-6 (around 10 balls total)

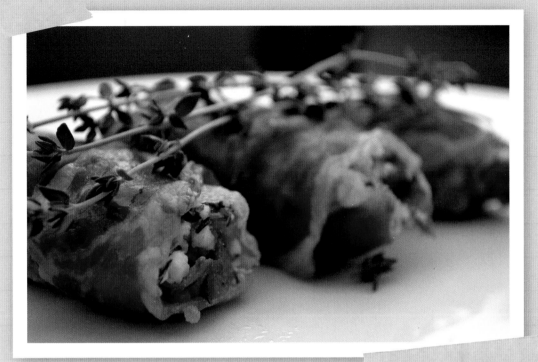

POCKETS OF POWER

These are great as either a quick snack or a side dish.

1 tablespoon olive oil,
   plus more for baking sheet
3 small sweet potatoes
1 tablespoon chopped fresh rosemary
1 teaspoon chopped thyme
2 ounces feta cheese or goat cheese
8-10 slices of prosciutto

PREPARATION TIME: 15 minutes
COOKING TIME: 10 minutes
SERVES: 4

1 Preheat oven to 350°F.

2 Add a little oil to a baking sheet to prevent the pockets from sticking.

3 Peel the sweet potatoes and chop them into cubes. Place into a steamer and cook until soft.

4 Place the rosemary and thyme into a bowl, and crumble in the feta or goat cheese, using a fork to blend them together. Once the sweet potatoes are cooked, mash them together with the cheese and herbs.

5 Now that your mixture is ready, place a slice of prosciutto into your hand and fill it with the sweet potato mixture. Do not pile in too much filling as you'll need to be able to roll up the prosciutto neatly.

6 Wrap up the ham and filling into a little parcel and place on the prepared baking sheet. Repeat with the remaining slices. Drizzle with olive oil and bake for 10 minutes or until the ham is nice and crispy on the edges.

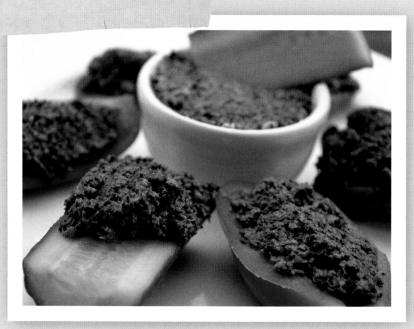

LIVER PÂTÉ

Liver is full of nutrients and one of the tastiest ways to eat it is blended into a pâté. Even if you aren't a liver lover, we reckon you'll enjoy this one.

2 tablespoons butter,
  plus more for the pan
6–8 slices of bacon, chopped into
  squares
2 garlic cloves, finely chopped
7 ounces mushrooms, sliced
½ pound chicken livers
Salt and pepper to taste

1 Melt the teaspoon of butter in a saucepan over low heat.

2 Add the bacon, garlic mushrooms, and chicken livers and cook for 8–10 minutes, until the chicken livers are browned.

3 Place all the ingredients in a food processor or blender, season to taste, and add the remaining butter. Blend into a pâté consistency.

4 Place in a dish lined with butter, and place in the fridge to cool until the fat hardens.

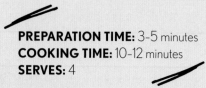

PREPARATION TIME: 3-5 minutes
COOKING TIME: 10-12 minutes
SERVES: 4

5 Enjoy as a snack on sliced cucumber, peppers, or beef tomatoes, or simply slice and enjoy on its own.

《TIP》 You can use either chicken or lamb's liver. For those who prefer a slightly milder tasting pâté, we recommend using chicken livers.

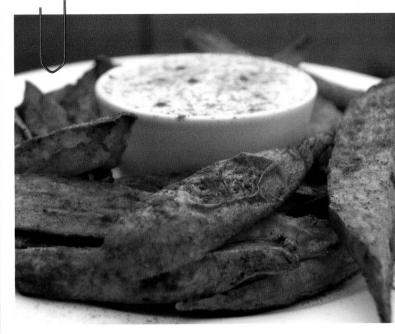

Sweet Potato Wedges

This awesome snack or side dish also tastes great with homemade Guacamole (page 174).

For the Wedges
4 large sweet potatoes
1 tablespoon coconut oil
3 teaspoons smoked paprika
1 teaspoon salt

For the Dipping Sauce
½ cup sour cream or crème fraîche
3 tablespoons chopped fresh chives
Dash of paprika

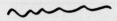

PREPARATION TIME: 5 minutes
COOKING TIME: 40-50 minutes
SERVES: 4

《TIP》

To make sweet potato chips, simply slice the potatoes into thin chip shapes and remove the chili.

1 Preheat the oven to 350°F.

2 Slice the sweet potatoes into 3- to 4-inch wedges.

3 Melt the coconut oil and mix in the smoked paprika and salt.

4 Coat the wedges in the oil and spices, and place on a baking sheet.

5 Bake for 40 minutes until soft yet lightly browned around the edges.

6 To make the dipping sauce, mix together the sour cream and chopped chives, sprinkle with paprika, and refrigerate until ready to serve.

7 Serve the hot wedges with the chive dipping sauce.

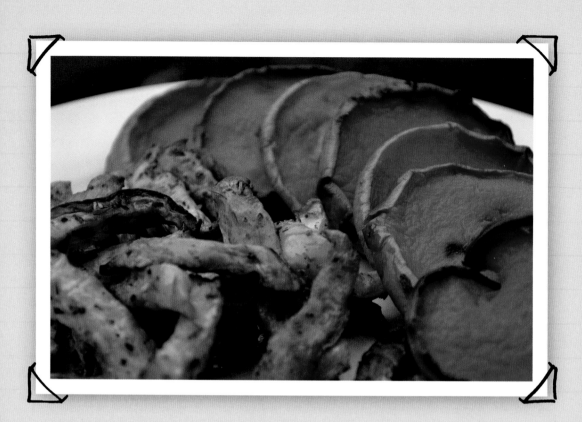

Baked Squash Discs

Roasted vegetables, especially root vegetables, are packed with vitamins and antioxidants and are a great source of energy. They make the perfect snack after you've been to the gym. You can even top them with some cooked meats for extra flavor.

1 whole butternut squash

《TIP》

Roasting large slices of just about any vegetables will work. We like sweet potato, parsnips, celeriac, or beetroot.

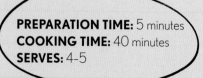

PREPARATION TIME: 5 minutes
COOKING TIME: 40 minutes
SERVES: 4-5

1 Preheat oven to 325°F.

2 Slice the whole squash, starting with the pointed end, into ½-inch-thick discs. As you get to the bulbous part containing the seeds, simply discard them from the middle of the squash.

3 Grease a large baking sheet or line it with parchment paper.

4 Lay the slices of squash across the baking sheet and bake for 40 minutes to an hour.

6 The skin should be slightly crispy while the flesh remains soft. These will keep for a couple of days.

Zucchini and Chive Fritters

Technically mini zucchini omelets, these are perfect as quick snacks any time of the day.

6 eggs
2 zucchinis, grated
Large handful of fresh chives, chopped
Coconut oil for the pan
Salt and pepper to taste

PREPARATION TIME: 4 minutes
COOKING TIME: 4 minutes
SERVES: 2

1 Beat the eggs in a large bowl.

2 Add the zucchini and half the chives into the eggs. Mix until smooth.

3 Heat a large pan over medium heat and add the butter or coconut oil.

4 Place 2-3 tablespoons of the mixture into the pan. Heat for 1-2 minutes and then flip over. They should be nice and golden on both sides.

5 Once cooked, season with salt and pepper and serve with the remaining chives.

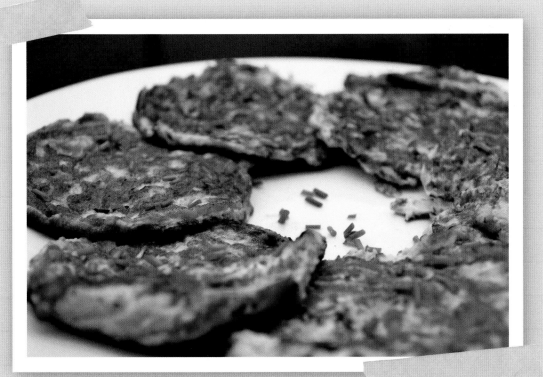

OUR TOP BURGER BITES

Burger King and Queen

Burgers are a big feature in our diet. They make such a tasty, convenient meal or snack any time of the day. Plus, ground meat is often cheaper to buy than whole cuts of meat. Just try to source the grass-fed variety from a trusted butcher. After that, it's great fun exploring different combinations of meats and herbs. We often compete for the best burger recipe.

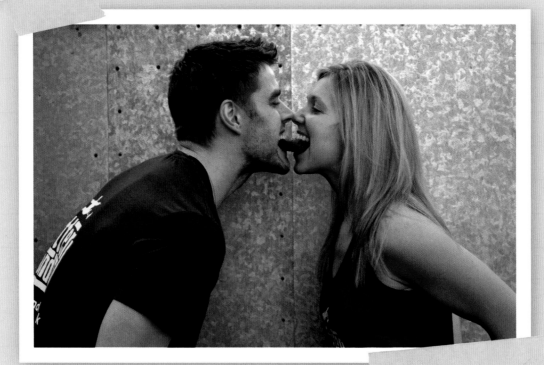

Everyone who knows me knows I'm a red meat man. My burgers of choice are usually beef, lamb, or wild meats like zebra, wagyu beef, and camel. (Don't knock it until you've tried it.) Stronger tasting meats are really complemented with more distinctive flavors such as garlic, onions, chili, mustard, or tomato.

I'm a huge fan of turkey or chicken burgers. Although poultry isn't a strong tasting meat, you can infuse it with lots of fresh herbs. Tarragon, rosemary, and thyme are a great addition—also try adding some Thai spices or Italian herb mixes.

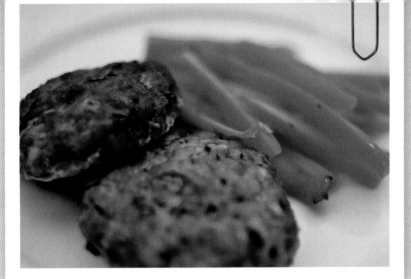

TARRAGON TURKEY BURGERS AND CITRUS FRIES

Lots of us love a roast turkey, but cooking with ground turkey can be a little trickier as it doesn't have the same juicy flavors as a big oven-roasted bird. We add lots of tarragon to turbo-boost the taste of a turkey burger, not to mention pack in some fantastic antioxidants.

For the Citrus Fries
4-5 carrots
Juice of half a lemon
4 garlic cloves, finely chopped

For the Burgers
1 pound ground turkey
1 egg
Large bunch of fresh tarragon, chopped

Serve with
Homemade Mayonnaise
(page 173)

PREPARATION TIME: 5 minutes
COOKING TIME: 40 minutes
SERVES: Makes 4-5 burgers

1 Preheat oven to 350°F.

2 Peel the carrots and slice them into thin fries.

3 Place the carrots on a baking sheet, squeeze the lemon juice over them, and sprinkle with half the garlic.

4 Bake for 40 minutes or until tender.

5 While the carrots are cooking, place the ground turkey in a large bowl and add the egg, the remaining garlic, and the tarragon. Using clean hands, mix all the ingredients together and shape into burger patties.

6 Place the patties on a grill pan and bake for 20-25 minutes. Once cooked, serve the burgers with the citrus carrot fries.

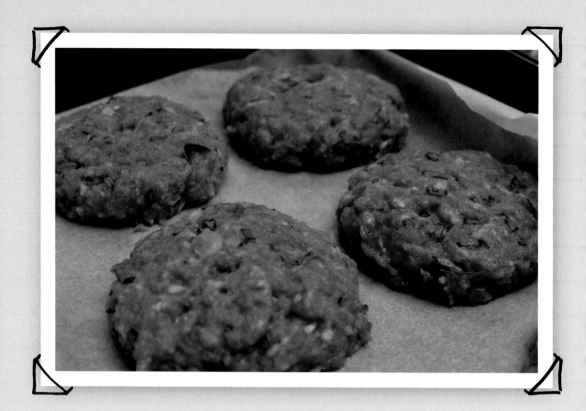

THAI BURGERS

Ground pork, chicken, or turkey all work with this Thai-style combination of lime, chili, and cilantro.

1 pound ground pork, chicken, or turkey
1 tablespoon fish sauce (optional)
1 egg
Juice of 1 lime
2 garlic cloves, finely chopped
Large handful of fresh cilantro, chopped
1 fresh green chili, chopped
Salt and pepper to taste

1 Preheat oven to 350°F.

2 Using clean hands, combine the meat, fish sauce, egg, lime juice, garlic, cilantro, chili, salt, and pepper in a large bowl.

3 Shape the mixture into burger patties, and place on a grill tray.

4 Bake for 20-25 minutes.

Serve with
Some bok choy sautéed in coconut oil

PREPARATION TIME: 5 minutes
COOKING TIME: 20-25 minutes
SERVES: Makes 4-5 burgers

Pesto Pork Cupcakes

These meaty cupcakes are a bit of fun, making them great for appetizers and party food. We use a dairy-free raw pesto called Seggiano in this recipe, but if you're OK with dairy, any organic brand will do. Dairy-free or otherwise, pesto is a simple, easy way to enhance the flavor of any kind of burger recipe.

1 pound ground pork (or you can use ground turkey or chicken)
2 tablespoons basil pesto
1 egg
Salt and pepper to taste

For the Topping
Butternut Smash (page 157)
8-10 cherry tomatoes

1 Preheat oven to 350°F.

2 Mix the meat, pesto, egg, salt and pepper in a large bowl with clean hands. Roll into a ball and mold to form a cupcake shape. Alternatively, you can shape the meat into standard burger patties.

3 Place the meat on a grill pan and bake for 20-25 minutes.

4 Once cooked, top with a teaspoon of Butternut Smash and a cherry tomato.

PREPARATION TIME: 5 minutes
COOKING TIME: 20-25 minutes
SERVES: Makes 8-10 cupcakes

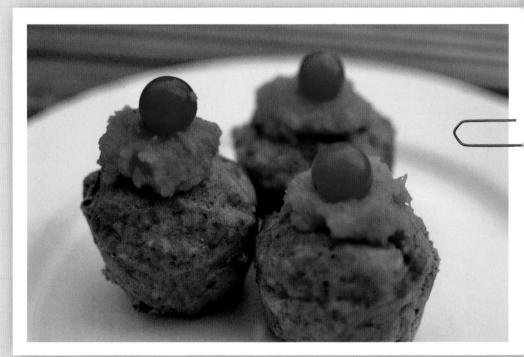

Turkey, Chestnut, and Rosemary Burgers

Chestnuts provide a good source of natural carbohydrates. We like to use chestnut flour for baking and add whole chestnuts to roasted vegetables, stuffing, or of course burgers!

1 pound ground turkey
1 egg
2 garlic cloves, finely chopped
6 sprigs of fresh rosemary, chopped
Salt and pepper to taste
1 cup peeled and roasted chestnuts

1 Preheat oven to 350°F.

2 In a large bowl, combine the ground turkey, egg, garlic, rosemary, salt, and pepper.

3 Chop the chestnuts and add them to the mixture.

4 Using clean hands, mix all the ingredients together and shape the mixture into burger patties.

5 Place on a grill pan and bake for 20 minutes.

PREPARATION TIME: 5 minutes
COOKING TIME: 20 minutes
SERVES: Makes 8 burgers

Serve with
Butternut Smash (page 157)

Lamb and Cumin Burgers

Lamb tastes great infused with blends of spices like cumin, smoked paprika, and ground coriander. In this recipe, we use cumin, garlic, and tomato paste, but you can try experimenting with your own spice mixes, too.

1 pound ground lamb
1 egg
3 garlic cloves, finely chopped
1 teaspoon ground cumin
3 tablespoons tomato paste
Salt and pepper to taste

1 Preheat oven to 350°F.

2 In a large bowl, combine the ground lamb, egg, garlic, cumin, tomato paste, salt, and pepper.

3 Using clean hands, mix all the ingredients together and shape into burger patties.

4 Place on a grill pan and bake for 20-25 minutes.

PREPARATION TIME: 5 minutes
COOKING TIME: 20-25 minutes
SERVES: Makes 4-5 burgers

Serve with
Steamed spinach and Chunky Zucchini Fries (page 162)

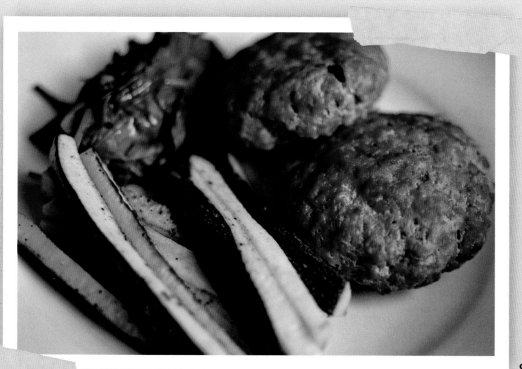

Matt's Big Beefy Onion and Chorizo

A simply mind-blowing combination!

1 pound ground beef
2 small chorizo sausages, chopped into
    bite-size cubes
1 egg
2 tablespoons tomato paste
½ red onion, peeled and finely
chopped
Salt and pepper to taste

1 Preheat oven to 350°F.

2 Place the ground beef in a large bowl. Using clean hands, combine with the chorizo, egg, tomato paste, and chopped onion.

3 Shape the mixture into burger patties and place on a grill tray.

4 Bake for 20-25 minutes.

PREPARATION TIME: 5 minutes
COOKING TIME: 20-25 minutes
SERVES: Makes 4-5 burgers

Serve with
Sweet Potato Wedges (page 89)

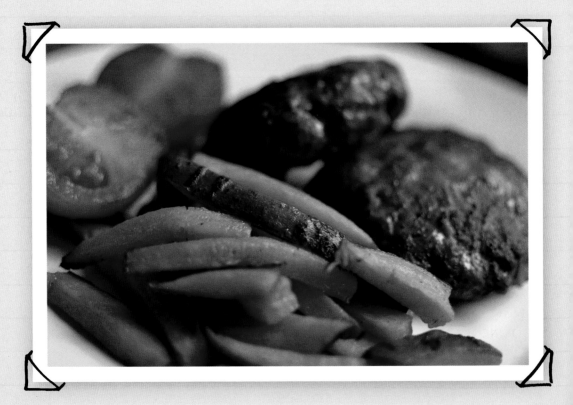

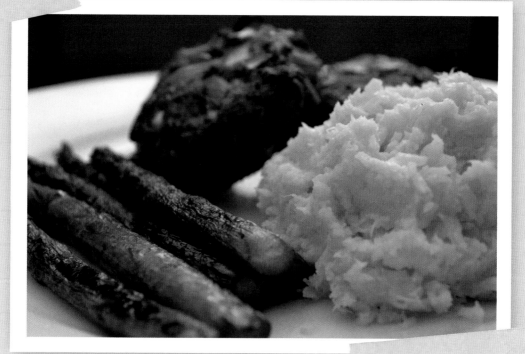

BEEF AND MUSTARD BURGERS

Roast beef and mustard chips are a favorite in the UK. We've made this winning flavor combination one our favorite burgers instead!

1 pound ground beef
1 egg
1 heaping tablespoon mustard powder
1 tablespoon chopped parsley
Salt and pepper to taste

Serve with
Cauliflower Mash (page 155)

1 Preheat oven to 350°F.

2 Using clean hands, combine all the ingredients in a large bowl. Shape the mixture into burger patties.

3 Place the patties on a grill pan and bake for 20-25 minutes.

PREPARATION TIME: 5 minutes
COOKING TIME: 20-25 minute
SERVES: Makes 4-5 burgers

Meals in Minutes

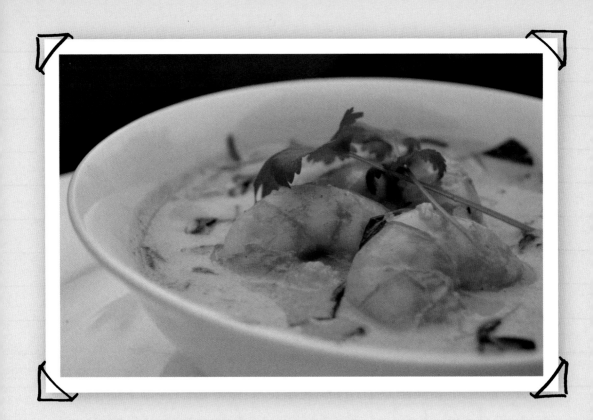

COCONUT COMFORT CURRY

Creamy, hot, and spicy. It's the perfect dish for miserable Monday nights. Ready in 10 minutes and full of antioxidant-rich herbs and spices to help you recover from the weekend.

1 14-ounce can of organic coconut milk
2 teaspoons curry powder
1 teaspoon grated fresh ginger
Coconut oil or ghee for the pan
1 onion, chopped
1 pound raw shrimp
2 large handfuls of fresh spinach
Fresh cilantro for garnish

1 Prepare the sauce by mixing together the coconut milk, curry powder, and grated ginger in a bowl. Set aside.

2 Stir-fry the onions in coconut oil or ghee for 2 minutes. Add the coconut curry sauce to the onions and simmer for 5 minutes.

3 Add the shrimp to the curry sauce and cook until pink.

4 Finally, add the spinach and allow it to wilt down. Garnish with the cilantro and serve.

PREPARATION TIME: 10 minutes
COOKING TIME: 10 minutes
SERVES: 4

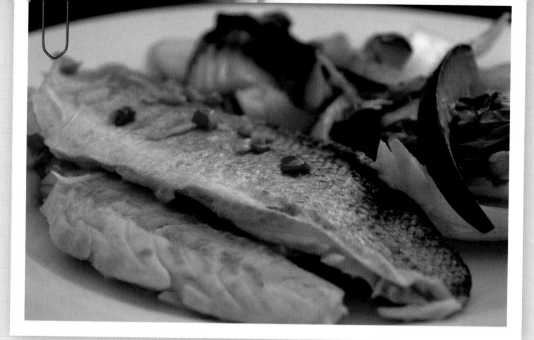

Thai Sea Bass Supper

No messing, no marinating—just a quick and easy way to infuse sea bass with tantalizing Thai flavors in 5 minutes.

Coconut oil for the pan
½ chili, chopped (use a whole chili if you like an extra kick)
3 garlic cloves, finely chopped
Large handful of fresh cilantro
1-inch piece of fresh ginger, peeled and grated
1 medium bok choy, chopped
1 zucchini, sliced
2 sea bass fillets
Juice of 1 lime
Salt and pepper to taste

1 Melt the coconut oil in a frying pan over low heat.

2 Add chili, garlic, cilantro, and ginger to the oil and stir-fry for 1 minute.

3 Add chopped bok choy and sliced zucchini to the pan, and toss to coat with the oil and spices.

4 Push the bok choy and zucchini to the side of the pan.

5 Place the sea bass in the pan skin side down, and after 2-3 minutes gently flip over the fish using a spatula.

6 Heat until fish is cooked through.

7 Squeeze the lime juice over the fish and vegetables, season with salt and pepper, and serve.

PREPARATION TIME: 5 minutes
COOKING TIME: 5 minutes
SERVES: 2

Serve with
Cauliflower Rice (page 154).

Sweet Garlic Shrimp

This is another great supper in seconds. The key ingredient is the creamed coconut bar, which adds a hint of sweetness to the garlic sauce.

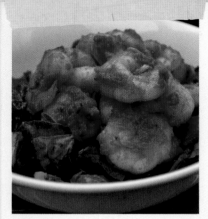

1 Melt the coconut oil over low heat.

2 Add chopped garlic and sauté for 2 minutes. Once the garlic starts to brown, add the raw shrimp. As soon as they start to change color, add the tomato sauce.

3 Grate the creamed coconut over the shrimp, and continue stirring until a creamy sauce starts to form.

4 Taste, and once you're happy with the sauce's consistency, serve the dish with steamed broccoli or a large mixed salad.

PREPARATION TIME: 5 minutes
COOKING TIME: 6 minutes
SERVES: 2

Coconut oil for the pan
2 garlic cloves, finely chopped
6 ounces raw shrimp, thawed
    (ideally wild, usually in the frozen section
    of supermarkets)
2-3 tablespoons Tomato Sauce
    (page 175 or store-bought)
1 tablespoon creamed coconut, grated
    from a block

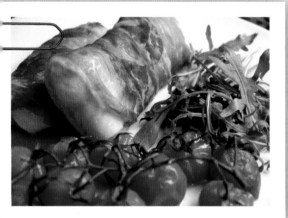

10 cherry tomatoes on the vine
2 garlic cloves, finely chopped
2 5-ounce whitefish fillets
1 tablespoon basil pesto
4 slices of prosciutto

PREPARATION TIME: 5 minutes
COOKING TIME: 20 minutes
SERVES: 2

Fish in a Blanket

Whitefish is often difficult to get excited about. Pesto and prosciutto are a couple of quick ways to add flavor. The garlic-roasted cherry tomatoes add even more punch.

1 Preheat oven to 350°F.

2 Place the tomatoes in a baking dish and sprinkle with the garlic; allow to roast for 20 minutes.

3 Meanwhile, brush each fillet with pesto and wrap with two slices of prosciutto .

4 Place the fillets on a baking sheet and bake for 12-15 minutes until cooked to your liking.

Serve with
Fresh arugula

Pan-Fried Spicy Mackerel

Mackerel is a fantastic source of essential omega-3 fats, and it's cheaper than most fish! Many people aren't too keen on the strong taste of mackerel, so combining it with spices like cumin and black pepper makes the fish taste a little milder.

2 5-ounce mackerel fillets
2 tablespoons apple cider vinegar
1 teaspoon ground cumin
½ teaspoon black pepper
2 pats of butter

PREPARATION TIME: 5 minutes
COOKING TIME: 20 minutes
SERVES: 2

1 Preheat oven to 350°F.

2 Place the mackerel fillets in a baking dish, topping each one with a tablespoon of apple cider vinegar and sprinkling with cumin and pepper. Then place a pat of butter (about a teaspoon) onto each fillet.

3 Bake the mackerel for around 20 minutes.

Serve with
Steamed spinach and Cauliflower Rice (page 154)

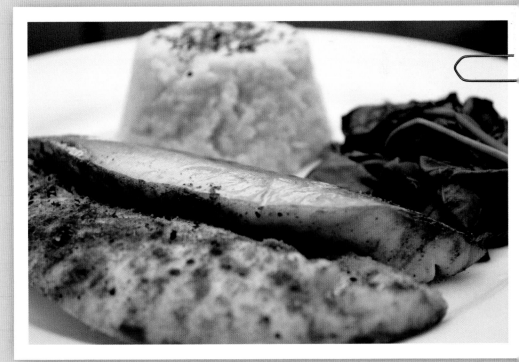

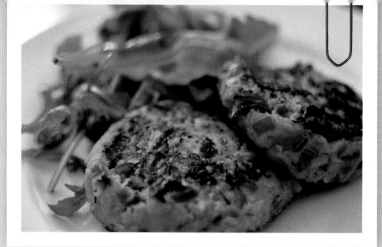

MACKEREL AND SWEET POTATO FISH CAKES

Another great way to boost your essential omega-3 fats. The sweet potato provides a milder tasting mackerel, so even if think you're not a fan of the fish, you may well become one!

2 small sweet potatoes
4 teaspoons coconut oil or butter
1 red onion, chopped
1 tablespoon fresh rosemary, chopped
2 peppered mackerel fillets, cooked
Salt and pepper

1 Chop the sweet potato into small chunks, place in a steamer, and cook until soft.

2 Melt half the coconut oil in a frying pan, gently cook the onion in it, and remove from the heat.

3 Drain the sweet potato and mash until smooth and creamy. Add the chopped rosemary.

4 Break up the fillets, and add them into the mashed sweet potato. Mix in the cooked onion.

5 Form the mixture into fish cakes.

6 Melt the remaining coconut oil in a frying pan and place the fish cakes on the heated pan.

7 After around 5 minutes, flip the cakes over. These only take a few minutes on each side, so you need to keep your eye on the pan and be ready to turn them. They are ready when both sides are a nice golden brown.

Serve with
A large mixed salad

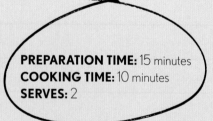

PREPARATION TIME: 15 minutes
COOKING TIME: 10 minutes
SERVES: 2

TIP
You can also make these with Butternut Smash (page 157) instead of sweet potatoes.

MUSTARD SEED SALMON

Mustard seeds are a true superfood and, in our opinion, not used enough. They have been studied repeatedly for their anti-cancer effects and ability to inhibit the growth of cancer cells. This combination of spices, seeds, and coconut is great with any fish or poultry.

Ghee or coconut oil for the pan
2 teaspoons white mustard seeds
¼ teaspoon fennel seeds (optional)
7 ounces coconut milk
¼ teaspoon ground cumin
¼ teaspoon ground turmeric
1 tablespoon English mustard powder
2 fresh chilies, chopped
   or 1 teaspoon chili powder
1 zucchini, sliced
3 5-ounce salmon fillets

1 Heat the ghee or oil in a medium-size frying pan.

2 Add the mustard seeds and stir-fry. Once they begin to pop, add the fennel seeds and pour in the coconut milk.

3 Add the cumin, turmeric, mustard powder, and chopped chilies or chili powder.

4 Add the sliced zucchini.

5 Bring the sauce to a gentle simmer and then add the fish.

6 Cook for an additional 5 minutes or until the fish is cooked through.

PREPARATION TIME: 10 minutes
COOKING TIME: 20 minutes
SERVES: 2

Serve with
Steamed vegetables

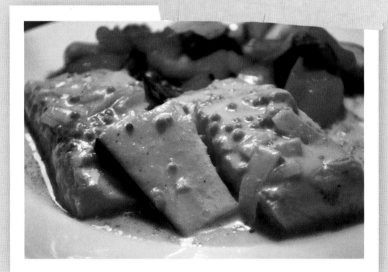

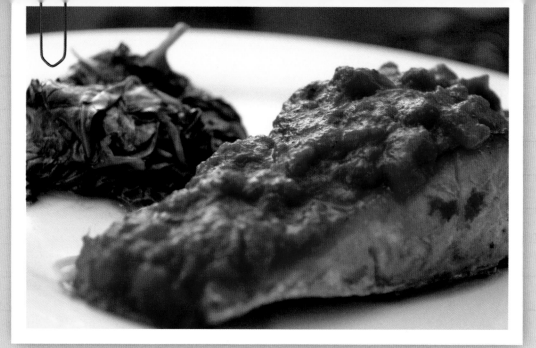

Baked Tomato Salmon

You won't believe how tasty this dish is, given how simple it is to prepare. The combination of spices does all the culinary work. This recipe also provides a fantastic range of antioxidants and our favorite anti-cancer spices: turmeric, black pepper, cumin, and garam masala.

Ghee or butter for the pan
1 red pepper, chopped
1 teaspoon turmeric
1 teaspoon black pepper
1 teaspoon ground cumin
1 teaspoon garam masala
Pinch of salt
4 5-ounce salmon fillets
1 cup or so of water or stock
1 tablespoon lemon juice
1 cup Tomato Sauce (page 175 or
    store-bought)

1 Add oil to a saucepan and sauté the chopped pepper and all the spices until the pepper softens.

2 Add the salmon fillets to the pan and pour in the tomato sauce and water or stock until the fish is completely covered.

3 Simmer over low heat for 5-8 minutes or until the salmon has cooked through.

4 Add lemon juice and serve.

Serve with
Chunky Zucchini Fries (page 162), or simply toss some spinach and kale into the sauce before serving.

PREPARATION TIME: 5 minutes
COOKING TIME: 15 minutes
SERVES: 4

Caribbean Jerk Salmon

Jerk seasoning can really transform any fish or meat. Even if you aren't a big fish lover, we bet you'll clear your plate.

1 teaspoon allspice
½ teaspoon cinnamon
½ teaspoon ground cumin
1 teaspoon smoked paprika
1 teaspoon cayenne or chili powder
1 teaspoon salt
2-inch piece of fresh ginger, peeled
   and finely chopped
2 garlic cloves, finely chopped
(or 1 teaspoon garlic powder)
2 tablespoons olive oil or coconut oil
Juice of 1 lime
4 5-ounce salmon fillets
Fresh cilantro for garnish

1 Preheat oven to 350°F.

2 Mix all the ingredients except the salmon in a bowl. If using coconut oil, be sure to melt it first. Keep mixing until all ingredients are blended together nicely.

3 Coat the salmon fillets in the marinade and place in a baking dish.

4 Top the salmon with any remaining marinade and place it in the oven.

5 Bake for 20-25 minutes, depending on how well you like your fish cooked. This tastes great if you allow the salmon to crisp on top.

6 Garnish with cilantro.

Serve with
Cauliflower Rice (page 154) or half an avocado for a healthy meal packed with good fats

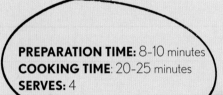

PREPARATION TIME: 8-10 minutes
COOKING TIME: 20-25 minutes
SERVES: 4

《TIP》

As with all marinades, this tastes best when prepared in advance and the salmon is left to marinate for 2-3 hours, or even better for 24 hours.

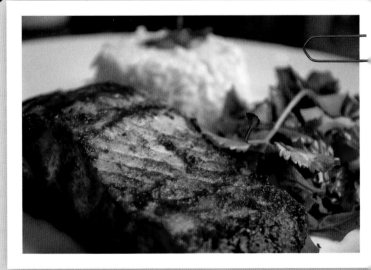

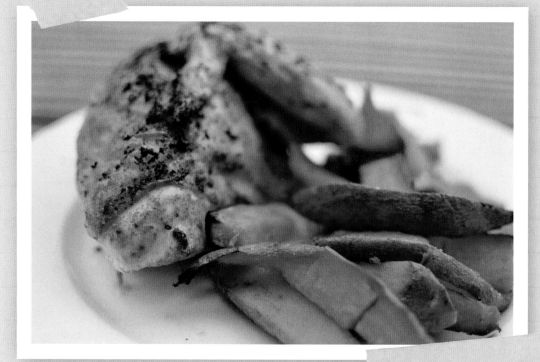

Quick Piri Piri Chicken

An instant take on a classic Portuguese favorite using just ghee and spices to flavor the chicken. No prizes for technicality here.

Ghee or butter for the pan
1 tablespoon chili powder
Zest of 1 lemon
4 garlic cloves, finely chopped
1 4-pound chicken, quartered

1 Preheat oven to 350°F.

2 Melt the ghee or butter and mix with the chili powder, lemon zest, and garlic.

3 Gently coat the chicken pieces with the oil and spices.

4 Place in a baking dish and bake for 40-50 minutes, until the juices run clear.

 TIP

Cook a whole chicken and turn the leftovers into lunch, as this tastes great cold with a large mixed salad.

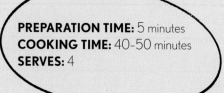

PREPARATION TIME: 5 minutes
COOKING TIME: 40-50 minutes
SERVES: 4

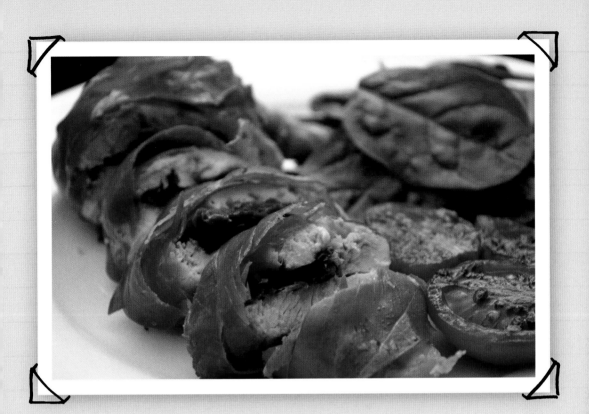

Sun-Dried Stuffed Chicken Breast

No messing, no marinating—just a quick and easy way to infuse chicken with some yummy Italian flavors in only minutes.

2 large boneless chicken breasts
4 Sun-Dried Tomatoes
   (page 168)
4 green olives, sliced
10–20 fresh basil leaves
6 slices of prosciutto

PREPARATION TIME: 5 minutes
COOKING TIME: 25 minutes
SERVES: 2

1 Preheat oven to 350°F.

2 Slice the raw chicken breast in half and place two sun-dried tomatoes, two sliced olives, and three to four torn basil leaves in between each breast.

3 Wrap each breast with three slices of prosciutto to seal the filling in place.

4 Place on a baking sheet and bake for 25 minutes.

Serve with
Fresh spinach salad and grilled tomatoes

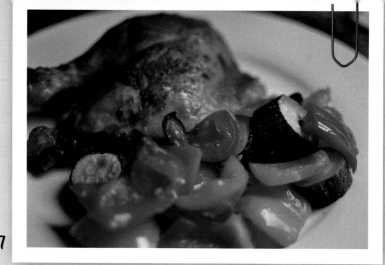

TURMERIC AND BLACK PEPPER CHICKEN WITH RAINBOW VEG

An awesome combination of great tasting spices and medicinal benefits. Turmeric and black pepper together have been shown to have powerful anti-cancer properties.

Ghee or butter for the pan
1 tablespoon ground turmeric
1 teaspoon black pepper
2 chicken breasts or 4 thighs/legs
2 garlic cloves, finely chopped
1 large onion, chopped
Pinch of salt
1 yellow or red pepper, chopped
8-10 cherry tomatoes
1 zucchini, sliced
Juice of half a lemon

1 Preheat oven to 350°F.

2 Melt 1 tablespoon of ghee or other oil. Place in a bowl and mix with the turmeric and black pepper.

3 Gently coat the chicken pieces with the oil and spices. Place the chicken in a baking dish and cook for 20-30 minutes.

4 Melt the rest of the oil in a frying pan over low heat. Add the garlic and onion and stir-fry.

5 Place chopped pepper, cherry tomatoes, sliced zucchini in the pan and toss in the oil, garlic, and salt.

6 Stir-fry until the peppers and zucchini begin to soften.

7 Serve the cooked chicken and vegetables together, squeezing the lemon juice over both.

PREPARATION TIME: 10 minutes
COOKING TIME: 20-30 minutes
SERVES: 2

THAI CHICKEN AND SCALLION RICE

This dish is so quick that you'll have no excuse for ordering out. Simple ingredients combine to make a fantastic tasting dish. Make extra and have the leftovers for lunch.

3 scallions
1 tablespoon coconut oil
1 heaping tablespoon Chinese five spice
1 garlic clove, finely chopped
½-inch piece of fresh ginger, peeled and finely chopped
2 large chicken breasts (keep skins on)

For the Rice
1 cup Cauliflower Rice (page 154)
Salt and pepper to taste

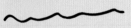

PREPARATION TIME: 5 minutes
COOKING TIME: 25 minutes
SERVES: 2

1 Preheat oven to 350 °F.

2 Chop the scallions. (These are for adding to the Cauliflower Rice, so set them aside.)

3 Melt the coconut oil and place in a medium bowl. Add the Chinese five spice, garlic, and ginger, and stir into a paste.

4 Coat the chicken in the marinade, and place the chicken pieces into a baking dish.

5 Bake the chicken for around 25-30 minutes, until cooked through. (Check by inserting a sharp knife; the juices should run clear.)

6 Five minutes before the chicken is ready, start to make the Cauliflower Rice and add the chopped scallions to the recipe. Cook the rice over low heat, stirring occasionally to prevent the cauliflower from overcooking.

7 Season the cauliflower with salt and pepper, and serve when chicken is ready.

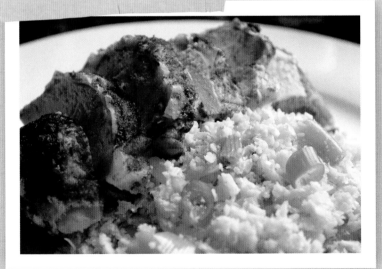

Everyday Chicken Curry

You might think preparing a curry will take hours, but this tasty, simple blend of spices with chopped tomatoes is incredibly quick to make and any meat or fish can be substituted.

Ghee, butter, or coconut oil for the pan
2 chicken breasts or 4 thighs/legs, chopped
2 teaspoons medium curry powder
2 teaspoons ground coriander
½ teaspoon ground cumin
½ teaspoon turmeric
½ teaspoon black pepper (optional)
1 tablespoon peeled and grated ginger
2 garlic cloves, finely chopped
1 large onion, chopped
1 14.5-ounce can of diced tomatoes

Serve with
Cauliflower Rice (page 154)

1 Add the oil to a saucepan and sauté the chicken for 5 minutes.

2 Add all the spices, ginger, garlic, onion, and tomatoes, until the chicken is covered. (Add extra water if needed.)

3 Bring to a boil and simmer for around 20-30 minutes or until the chicken is cooked and tender.

PREPARATION TIME: 10 minutes
COOKING TIME: 40 minutes
SERVES: 2

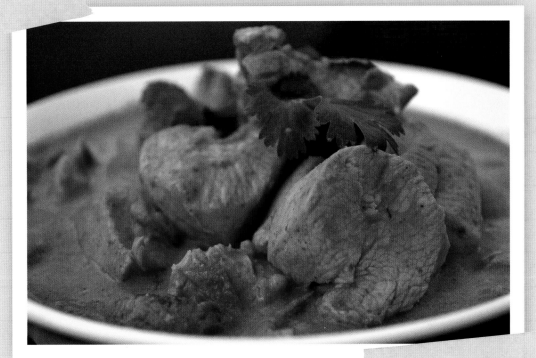

Turkey Coconut Curry

A quick and simple curry that's great for entertaining midweek.

1 13.5-ounce can of coconut milk
2 garlic cloves, finely chopped
½-inch piece of fresh ginger, peeled and
   finely chopped
1 tablespoon white mustard seeds
1 teaspoon ground cumin
1 tablespoon coriander powder
1 teaspoon ground turmeric
3 hot chilies or 1 teaspoon hot chili powder
2 onions, chopped
2-3 fresh tomatoes, quartered
7 ounces mushrooms (optional)
1 pound diced turkey

1 Combine coconut milk, garlic, ginger, mustard seeds, spices, chilies (or chili powder), onions, tomatoes, and mushrooms in a large saucepan. Simmer over low heat.

2 Add the diced turkey, adding water if needed so the sauce covers the meat.

3 Bring to a boil and simmer for around 20-30 minutes or until the turkey is cooked and tender.

Serve with
Cauliflower Rice (page 154)

PREPARATION TIME: 10 minutes
COOKING TIME: 20-30 minutes
SERVES: 2

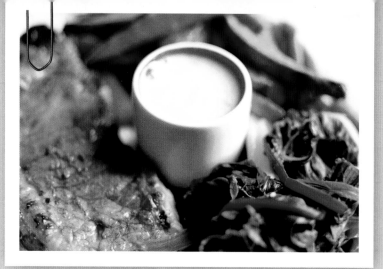

Grass-Fed Steak with Garlic Fries and Béarnaise Sauce

A healthy take on a classic favorite. This is usually our Friday night supper.

For the Garlic Fries
2 sweet potatoes, chopped into fries
2 garlic cloves, finely chopped
1 tablespoon butter or ghee

For the Béarnaise Sauce
3 egg yolks
2 tablespoons hot water
3 tablespoons olive oil
1 tablespoon lemon juice
Salt and pepper to taste

For the Steak
2 grass-fed steaks
1 tablespoon butter or ghee

Serve with steamed greens

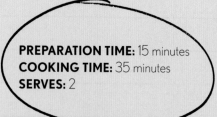

PREPARATION TIME: 15 minutes
COOKING TIME: 35 minutes
SERVES: 2

1 Preheat oven to 350°F.

2 Place the chopped sweet potato in a baking dish and top with the garlic and 1 tablespoon of butter or ghee. Bake for a few minutes, allowing the fat to melt, then toss the baking dish to ensure all the fries are coated in the garlic and oil. Bake for 25–30 minutes.

3 Meanwhile, make the béarnaise sauce. In a heat-proof bowl, gently whisk the egg yolks. Continue mixing and slowly add the hot water, olive oil, lemon juice, salt, and pepper.

4 Place the bowl over a saucepan of simmering water, fitted as a double boiler. Keep whisking until the sauce begins to thicken. (It shouldn't take long, around 30 seconds.) Then keep the sauce at room temperature.

5 When the fries are almost cooked, panfry the steak over low-medium heat in a tablespoon of butter or ghee, turning each minute until it is cooked to your liking.

6 Serve the steak and fries with the béarnaise sauce on the side.

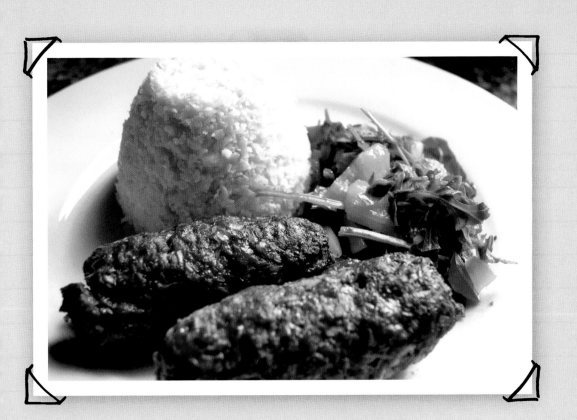

Lebanese-Style Beef

We love Lebanese food, and this dish is quick to prepare and packs a tasty punch. Delicious served warm from the oven, or enjoy the leftovers as a cold snack the next day.

1 pound ground beef
1 medium white onion, finely chopped
½ teaspoon cinnamon
½ teaspoon cayenne
½ teaspoon pepper
½ teaspoon ground cumin
½ teaspoon salt

1 Preheat oven to 350°F.

2 Place all the ingredients in a large bowl and mix together using your hands. Once all the ingredients have been blended, mold the mixture into sausage shapes.

3 Place on an baking sheet and cook for 15-20 minutes, turning after 10 minutes.

Serve with
Cauliflower Rice (page 154) and a green salad

PREPARATION TIME: 10 minutes
COOKING TIME: 15-20 minutes
SERVES: 2

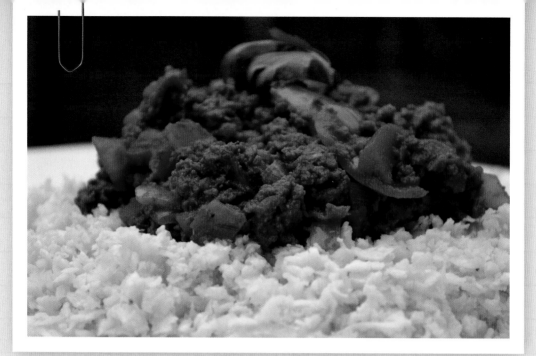

CHILI CON CAULIFLOWER

Who doesn't love chili—especially one that can be rustled up in just over half an hour? We cook a large batch as it always tastes better the next day and makes a great supper or snack.

Ghee or butter for the pan
2 pounds ground beef or lamb
2 red onions, cubed
3 tomatoes, cubed
2 tablespoons tomato paste
1 14-ounce can of chopped tomatoes
3 garlic cloves, finely chopped
1 red pepper, sliced
1 tablespoon mixed herbs
1 heaping teaspoon chili powder
1 tablespoon smoked paprika
1 tablespoon ground cumin
½ teaspoon salt
1 teaspoon pepper

For the Rice
Cauliflower Rice (page 154)

Try this topped with
Guacamole (page 174)

1 You can start by browning the ground meat and onions in a little oil. However, an even quicker option is to place all the ingredients in a large saucepan, mix together, cover, and gently simmer over low heat for 25-30 minutes.

2 While the chili cooks, prepare the Cauliflower Rice.

3 After 25 minutes, start tasting the mixture and decide whether you wish to add a little more herbs, chili, or seasoning.

4 Serve on a bed of Cauliflower Rice.

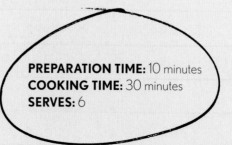

PREPARATION TIME: 10 minutes
COOKING TIME: 30 minutes
SERVES: 6

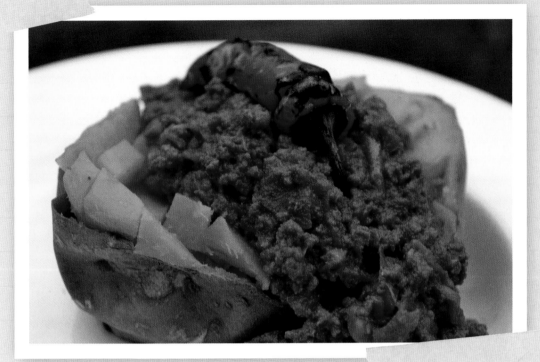

WHACK IT IN A SWEET POTATO JACKET

A nutrient-rich sweet potato jacket can be baked in roughly 40 minutes to an hour and topped with pretty much anything. Always have some leftovers ready to whack in a jacket.

* A can of tuna
* Sardines and fresh Ketchup (page 172)
* Mackerel and pan-fried mushrooms
* Egg with Homemade Mayonnaise (page 173)
* Chili (page 120) and sour cream

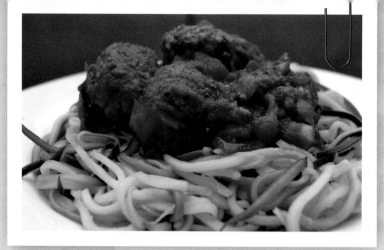

ITALIAN MEATBALLS

This is a classic Italian dish, but we've swapped the pasta for something more nutrient-dense: zucchini spaghetti. It's fantastic for a big family dinner. You will need a julienne peeler for this.

For the Meatballs
1 egg
1 pound ground beef
2 tablespoons finely chopped fresh
  rosemary
1 heaping tablespoon oregano
Salt and pepper to taste
Ghee or butter for the pan

For the Sauce
1 large white onion, chopped
6 black poplar mushrooms, chopped
4 garlic cloves, finely chopped
10-20 fresh basil leaves, finely chopped
2 14-ounce cans of chopped tomatoes
1 teaspoon chili powder (optional)

For the Spaghetti
3 zucchinis, julienned
  (see Vegetable Spaghetti,
  page 160)

`·  ·  ·  ·  ·  ·  ·  ·  ·`

PREPARATION TIME: 10 minutes
COOKING TIME: 20-25 minutes
SERVES: 4

`·  ·  ·  ·  ·  ·  ·  ·  ·`

1 Start by making the meatballs. In a large bowl, beat an egg and add the ground beef, oregano, chopped rosemary, salt and pepper. Use your hands to mix together thoroughly.

2 Melt some butter or ghee in a large pan. Shape the mixture into meatballs around 2 inches in diameter and place in the pan over medium heat, moving it around every now and then to ensure that the meat browns on all sides.

3 While these are cooking, start to make the sauce. In another large pan, heat the butter or ghee and add the onion, mushrooms, garlic, and basil.

4 Stir the ingredients and cook through until the onion and mushroom have softened slightly.

5 Add the tomatoes and chili powder, and stir. Bring the sauce to a simmer.

6 Add the meatballs to the sauce and continue to simmer for 5 minutes while you make the spaghetti.

7 To prepare the zucchini spaghetti, melt a little butter or ghee in a saucepan and add the julienned zucchini. (You can grate the zucchini if you don't have a julienne slicer.) Keep stirring until the zucchini softens to a texture you prefer.

8 Drain the spaghetti. Serve topped with the sauce and meatballs.

Lightning Lamb Kebabs

Why are these called Lightning Lamb Kebabs? Simply because they are so quick to prepare and cook. Lamb is one of our favorite meats, and this recipe is inspired by some of the great-tasting lamb dishes we tried during our vacation on the Greek island of Santorini. These lamb kebabs are great straight from the oven, but are so flavorsome they're awesome served cold the next day, too.

3 tablespoons olive oil
2 garlic cloves, finely chopped
1 tablespoon smoked paprika
1 teaspoon ground cumin
Salt and pepper to taste
1 pound lamb, cut into 1½-inch cubes
6-8 fresh sprigs of rosemary
   or kebab sticks
1 red pepper, deseeded and cut
   into 1-inch squares
1 red onion, peeled and quartered

1 Preheat grill to medium heat so it is ready as soon as the kebabs are prepared.

2 Mix the olive oil, garlic, smoked paprika, cumin, salt, and pepper together in a bowl until it turns into a paste.

3 Add the paste to the pieces of lamb and coat thoroughly.

4 Prepare the rosemary sprigs by removing a few of the leaves from the bottom of the sprig. Skewer the lamb, peppers, and onion onto the rosemary sprigs, alternating meat and vegetables. (Spear them at the base of the rosemary sprig, as this is much easier.)

5 Place the kebabs on the grill for 5-10 minutes, turning regularly until cooked to your liking.

PREPARATION TIME: 8-10 minutes
COOKING TIME: 10 minutes
SERVES: 2

Serve with
a large mixed salad

《TIP》

Marinate the lamb the day before for maximum taste, and use rosemary sprigs in place of wooden kebab sticks to add some extra Mediterranean flavor.

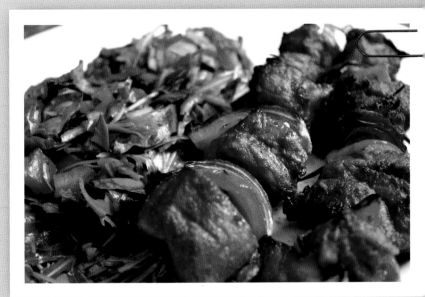

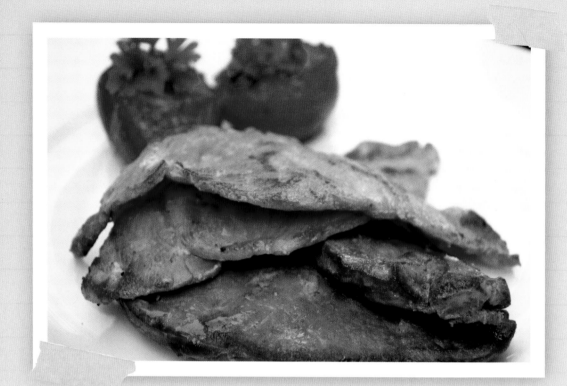

Liver and Bacon

Another attempt at getting this superfood into your weekly meals. This time we use bacon and cooked onions—with cooked tomatoes on the side—because you must love one of them.

Butter or ghee for the pan
½ onion, thinly sliced
2 slices of bacon
2 tomatoes, sliced
3-4 slices lamb's liver
Salt and pepper to taste

1 Melt the butter or ghee in a large frying pan, and cook the onions and bacon over low-medium heat, stirring frequently.

2 When the bacon is cooked through, add the sliced tomato to the pan.

3 When the tomato has softened, add the liver to the pan and cook for a few minutes on each side.

4 The liver is ready to serve when it's nicely browned on the outside, yet still pink and juicy on the inside.

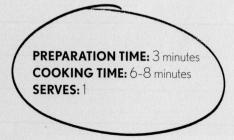

PREPARATION TIME: 3 minutes
COOKING TIME: 6-8 minutes
SERVES: 1

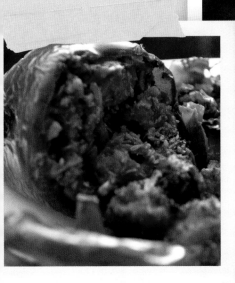
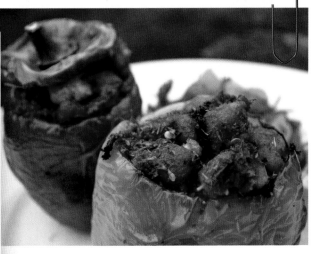

Sausage-Stuffed Peppers

An old vegetarian favorite converted into a meat and vegetable feast.

1 head of cauliflower, grated
Coconut oil for the pan
2 garlic cloves, finely chopped
1 red onion, peeled and chopped
6 assorted bell peppers
9 gluten-free sausages, chopped
10-20 fresh basil leaves, finely chopped
3 tablespoons tomato paste
1 teaspoon oregano
Salt and pepper to taste

- - - - - - - - -

PREPARATION TIME: 10 minutes
COOKING TIME: 30 minutes
SERVES: 4-6

- - - - - - - -

《 TIP 》

If you include dairy in your diet, try adding some quality goat cheese into the mixture before stuffing the pepper and baking.

1 Preheat oven to 350°F.

2 Melt a little coconut oil in a pan and add the crushed garlic.

3 Add the chopped onion and grated cauliflower and stir-fry for 5 minutes.

4 While the cauliflower and onion cook, gently remove the tops from the peppers and remove the stalks, seeds, and white fleshy parts.

5 Now add the sausages to the pan with the cauliflower, onion, and garlic. Keep stir-frying and mixing the ingredients together.

6 Add the tomato paste, fresh basil, oregano, salt and pepper.

7 Cook until the meat is browned and the onions are soft.

8 Spoon the mixture into the hollow peppers.

9 Place stuffed peppers in a baking dish, and bake for 30 minutes.

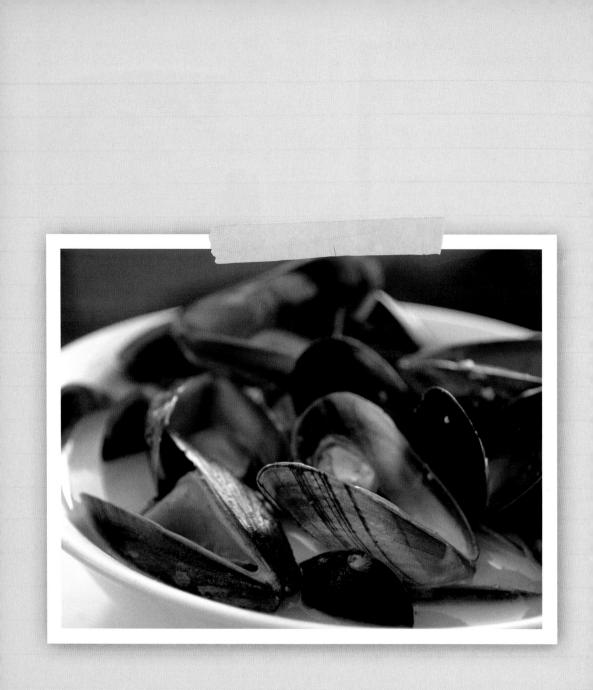

MUSSELS IN MINUTES

Mussels are usually pretty cheap, and they're so quick to prepare. Try to eat your mussels the same day you buy them. Fresh is always best with seafood.

MOULES MARINARA

2 pounds fresh mussels
1½ cup Tomato Sauce (page 175 or store-bought)
2 garlic cloves, finely chopped
¼ teaspoon chili powder (or more if you like it hot)
Fresh cilantro for garnish (optional)

~~~~~~

PREPARATION TIME: 10 minutes
COOKING TIME: 5-10 minutes
SERVES: 2

~~~~~~

1 To prepare the mussels, place them in cold water to wash and remove the beards (the hairy, stringy bit attached).

2 Place the clean mussels in a large saucepan and cover with tomato sauce, garlic, and chili powder.

3 Place the lid on the saucepan and steam the mussels over medium heat for 5-10 minutes until each one opens. Discard any mussels that do not open.

4 Sprinkle with cilantro and serve.

THAI MUSSELS

2 pounds fresh mussels
1 13.5-ounce can of coconut milk
1 garlic clove, crushed or finely chopped
2 kaffir lime leaves (available in Asian markets)
1 lemongrass stalk
¼ teaspoon chili powder
Fresh cilantro for garnish (optional)

~~~~~~

PREPARATION TIME: 10 minutes
COOKING TIME: 5-10 minutes
SERVES: 2

1 To prepare the mussels, place them in cold water to wash and remove the hairy, stringy beards attached.

2 Place the clean mussels in a large pan and cover with the coconut milk, garlic, lime leaves, lemongrass, and chili powder.

3 Place the lid on the pan and steam the mussels over medium heat for 5-10 minutes until each one opens. Discard any mussels that do not open.

4 Top with cilantro and serve.

Paleo comfort Food

MEDITERRANEAN BAKE

Add this to any meat and fish or simply enjoy as a meal in itself.

4 tablespoons olive oil
5 garlic cloves, finely chopped
1 small eggplant, cut into strips
1 sweet potato, cut into strips
2 white onions, peeled and thinly sliced
1 red pepper, thinly sliced
1 yellow pepper, thinly sliced
2 tablespoons mixed herbs
2 tablespoons parsley
Salt and pepper to taste
2 tomatoes, sliced
2 zucchinis, sliced
3½ ounces goat cheese
   (optional, but tastes amazing!)

1 Preheat oven to 350°F.

2 Heat 2 tablespoons of olive oil in a pan and add the crushed garlic. Stir-fry for a minute and then add the eggplant, sweet potato, onions, and peppers.

3 Continue to stir-fry and add salt and pepper, and half of the mixed herbs and half of the parsley.

4 Once sautéed, add vegetables to a baking dish and top with the sliced tomatoes, goat cheese, zucchini, and the remaining mixed herbs and parsley. Drizzle with another 2 tablespoons of olive oil and place in the oven.

5 Bake for 40-45 minutes and serve hot from the oven.

PREPARATION TIME: 15 minutes
COOKING TIME: 40-45 minutes
SERVES: 6

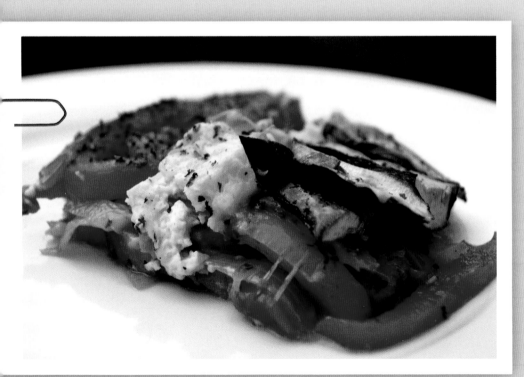

Primal Shepherd's Pie

Few things are as comforting on a cold, dark night than a hearty bowl of meat, herbs, and vegetables topped with creamy mash.

1 pound ground beef or lamb
2 white onions, chopped
2 medium-size carrots, sliced
3 garlic cloves, finely chopped
Macadamia oil, ghee, or butter
    for the pan
1 tablespoon chopped fresh rosemary
1 tablespoon chopped fresh thyme
2 teaspoons smoked paprika
2 heaping tablespoons tomato paste
Salt and pepper to taste

For the Topping
Cauliflower Mash (page 155),
double the recipe

1 Preheat oven to 350°F.

2 Heat oil in a pan and place the ground meat, onions, carrots, and garlic in the pan to brown.

3 Once the onions and carrots have softened and the meat has started to brown, mix in the fresh herbs, smoked paprika, tomato paste, salt and pepper. Let it heat through for another 5 minutes.

4 While the mixture is cooking, start to make the Cauliflower Mash topping. (Remember to double the recipe on page 155.)

5 Place the meat mixture into a 9 x 13-inch casserole dish and top with a one-inch layer of Cauliflower Mash. Cover the meat completely, not leaving any gaps.

6 Place in the oven and cook for 30-40 minutes until the topping browns nicely.

PREPARATION TIME: 15 minutes
COOKING TIME: 40 minutes
SERVES: 6

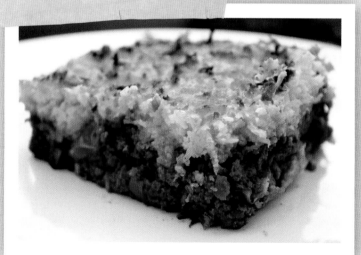

If you like more of a gravy with your Primal Pie, add a cup of meat stock to the meat filling before topping with the Cauliflower Mash.

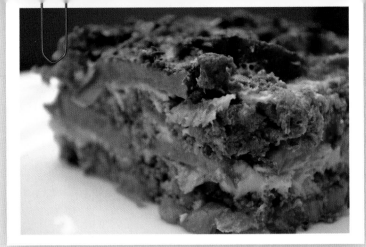

Man Maker Pie

Despite the name, have no fear, ladies—you can tuck into this truly phenomenal meal, too. The question is, "Are you man enough?"

5 medium sweet potatoes
6 slices of unsmoked bacon
2 pounds ground beef or lamb
4 garlic cloves, finely chopped
3 medium red onions
4 teaspoons smoked paprika
1-2 teaspoons cayenne chili
4 teaspoons oregano
2 tablespoons mixed herbs
3 heaping tablespoons tomato paste
12 eggs
Salt and pepper to taste

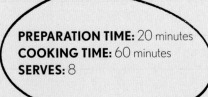

PREPARATION TIME: 20 minutes
COOKING TIME: 60 minutes
SERVES: 8

1 Preheat oven to 350°F.

2 Cut the sweet potatoes into ½-inch slices, chop the bacon into strips, and peel and slice the onions.

3 Cook the bacon in a frying pan over medium heat until browned slightly; remove from the pan and set aside.

4 Add the ground meat, garlic, and onions to the pan and stir-fry. Add the smoked paprika, cayenne chili, oregano, mixed herbs, and tomato paste. Continue to fry for an additional 10 minutes, stirring occasionally until the meat is browned and the onions have softened.

5 While the meat is cooking in the pan, prepare the eggs. Beat them in a large bowl, add a pinch of salt and pepper, and set aside.

6 Grease the base and sides of a 9 x 13-inch casserole dish (remember, the egg will rise a bit). Layer the dish several times over in the following order:
❋ Sweet potato slices
❋ Bacon, scattered
❋ Ground beef, onion, and spices

7 Repeat these layers until you have no ingredients left, then pour the beaten eggs over the top. Move the dish side to side to ensure the egg mixture fills in all the gaps. Place it in the oven and cook for 1 hour.

8 Serve hot from the oven, no sides necessary!

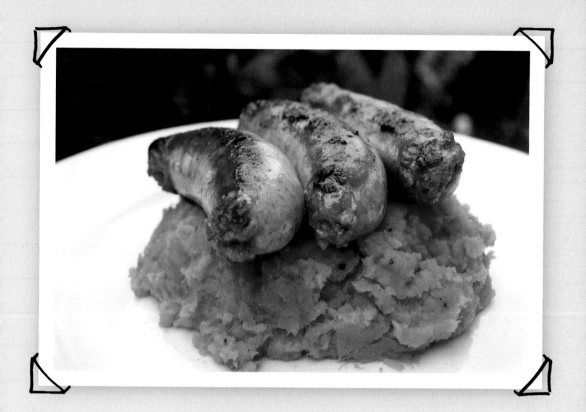

Bangers and Mash

Bangers and mash is easily one of the best British dishes around. Choose the mash based on your preference of cauliflower, parsnip, or sweet potato.

2 tablespoons butter or ghee, plus
   more for the pan
4 large gluten-free sausages
2 medium sweet potatoes, chopped
Salt and pepper to taste

Serve with
Buttered Savoy Cabbage (page 164)

PREPARATION TIME: 10 minutes
COOKING TIME: 20 minutes
SERVES: 2

1 Melt 1 teaspoon of butter or ghee in a saucepan over medium heat. Place the sausages in the pan and cook for 15 minutes or so, turning occasionally.

2 While the sausages are cooking, place the sweet potato in a steamer for about 10-15 minutes or until soft.

3 Once the potato is cooked, place in a bowl and add the butter or ghee. Mash with a fork or potato masher. Season to taste with salt and pepper.

4 Serve the sausages on the mashed sweet potatoes with a side of Buttered Savoy Cabbage; pour the fat from the sausages as a gravy.

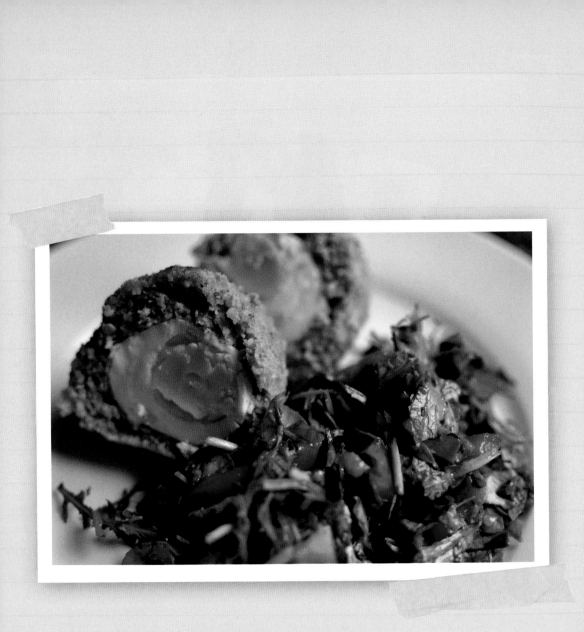

Matt's Mighty Scotch Egg

A family favorite, passed down through generations. Simply awesome!

14 eggs
12 gluten-free pork sausages, casings
   removed
3 tablespoons mixed herbs
Salt and pepper to taste
4 ounces ground almonds

PREPARATION TIME: 15 minutes
COOKING TIME: 30 minutes
SERVES: Makes 12 Scotch Eggs

1 Preheat the oven to 350°F.

2 Fill a saucepan with water enough to cover 12 eggs. Boil the eggs for 4 minutes.

3 Place the sausage meat, herbs, salt, and pepper in a large bowl, and mix thoroughly with your hands.

4 Remove the eggs from the saucepan and peel the shells off.

5 Beat the remaining two eggs in a bowl, and empty the ground almonds onto a plate.

6 Shape a handful of sausage meat around each hard-boiled egg. It is roughly one sausage per egg. Aim for a layer about ½ an inch thick.

7 Coat each sausage-wrapped egg in the beaten egg before rolling into the ground almonds.

8 Place the Scotch eggs on a baking sheet and bake for 30 minutes. Once it's baked, the almonds will create a crunchy coating.

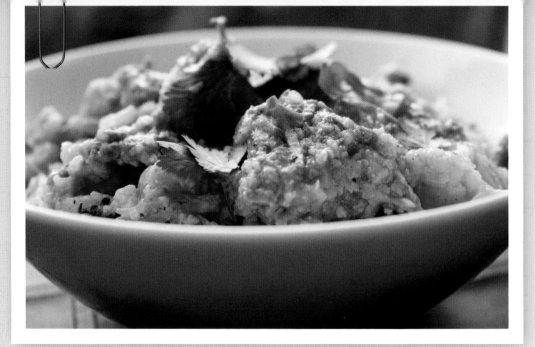

BEEF AND CREAMY CAULIFLOWER TAGINE

This dish is nothing short of phenomenal. The cauliflower disintegrates, leaving the spicy beef in a delicious creamy sauce. Try it once and we bet it will soon become a regular favorite of yours. This is a huge serving, so you can freeze the leftovers and reheat it as a quick supper during the week.

2 pounds grass-fed diced beef
   (stewing or braising steak)
1 red onion, chopped
1-2 tablespoons chopped cilantro
1½ teaspoon hot paprika
¼ teaspoon ginger powder
¼ teaspoon turmeric
1 teaspoon salt
2 medium cauliflowers, stems removed,
   and chopped into large florets
Fresh cilantro as garnish

1 Add beef, onion, spices, and salt to a large pan and cover with water.

2 Bring to a boil and gently simmer for 1 hour or until the meat is tender.

3 Add the cauliflower. Cook until all the cauliflower disintegrates and leaves a thickened sauce.

4 Serve in a large bowl topped with fresh cilantro.

PREPARATION TIME: 10 minutes
COOKING TIME: 1 hour 30 minutes
SERVES: 6-8

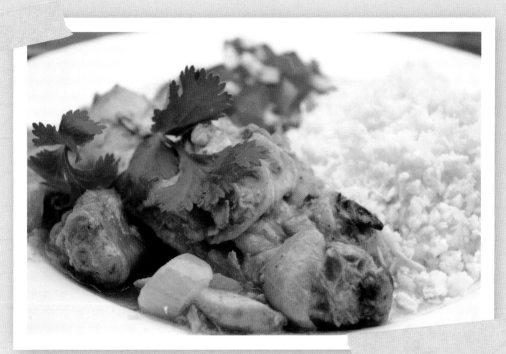

CHICKEN VINDALOO

Friday night curry is legendary in the UK. Who knew that it's also a pretty healthy dish?

6-8 chicken thighs
2 garlic cloves, finely chopped
1 onion, sliced
1 tablespoon curry powder
1 teaspoon cumin
1 teaspoon turmeric
1 teaspoon black pepper
1 tablespoon or so ground coriander,
    depending on your taste
1 teaspoon or so chili powder (add more
    or less for hotter or milder curry)
1 cup apple cider vinegar
Pinch of salt

Serve with
Cauliflower Rice (page 154)

1 Add the chicken thighs, garlic, onion, spices, vinegar, and salt to a large saucepan and cover with water.

2 Bring to a boil and simmer for around 40 minutes or until the liquid is reduced and the chicken is cooked and tender.

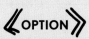

Use a whole chicken. Once the meat is tender, remove the chicken from the pan, strip the meat, and add back into the vindaloo sauce, discarding the skin and bones before serving.

PREPARATION TIME: 10 minutes
COOKING TIME: 40 minutes
SERVES: 2

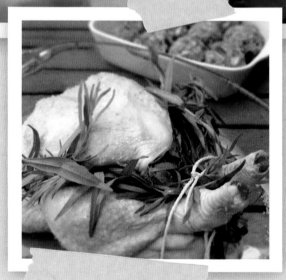

 TIP

Use your finger to separate the
skin from the breast, then stuff
fresh tarragon sprigs under
the skin. This way, the tarragon
imparts a great flavor.

Tarragon Roast Chicken and Chestnut Stuffing

This is a really simple way to infuse a roast chicken. Fresh tarragon is great with poultry, and as far as we're concerned, the more you stuff under the skin, inside, and around the meat, the better.

For the Chicken
1 whole free-range chicken
Large bunch of fresh tarragon
3-4 garlic cloves, finely chopped
2-3 whole garlic cloves
1 lemon
Salt and pepper to taste

For the Stuffing
1 pound ground pork
1 red onion, finely chopped
8 ounces peeled and roasted chestnuts, chopped
1 egg
1 tablespoon mixed herbs
Salt and pepper to taste

Serve with
Butternut Smash (page 157)

PREPARATION TIME: 10 minutes
COOKING TIME: 90 minutes
SERVES: 4

1 Preheat oven to 350°F.

2 Pierce the skin on the breasts and legs, and stuff with the tarragon and chopped garlic cloves.

3 Prick holes in the lemon with a knife and place inside the chicken with the rest of the fresh tarragon.

4 Bash the two whole garlic cloves with a jar, a can, or the flat side of a knife so that the skin breaks, and place the cloves inside the chicken with the lemon and tarragon.

5 Place the chicken on a roasting tray in the oven. It should take around 90 minutes to cook (double-check the cooking time based on the weight of the chicken).

6 Halfway through cooking, remove the chicken from the oven and baste it in its juices (take large spoonfuls of the juices in the tray and drizzle over the chicken).

7 Prepare the Butternut Smash.

8 For the stuffing, mix the ground pork with the chopped onions, chestnuts, egg, mixed herbs, salt, and pepper.

9 Flatten the stuffing mixture into a casserole dish. When the chicken is roughly 30 minutes from being cooked through, place the stuffing in the oven and bake until crispy on top.

10 Remove the chicken from the oven (keep the juices to use as gravy), cover, and allow to stand for 10-15 minutes.

11 Carve the tarragon chicken and serve with a large slab of stuffing and lots of Butternut Smash. For gravy, spoon over the juices from the cooked chicken.

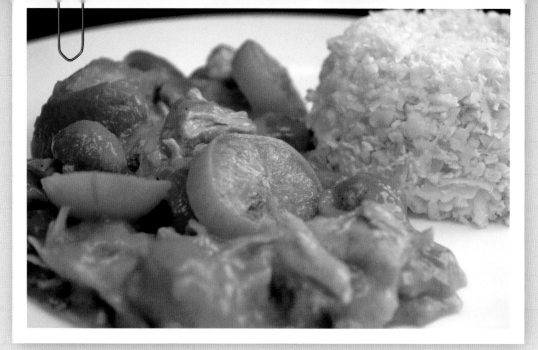

Lemon and Olive Chicken Tagine

This is a family favorite and it's great to serve when entertaining friends. We've yet to meet anyone who doesn't love this lemon-infused, spicy Moroccan dish.

1 whole free-range chicken
2 Preserved Lemons (page 176), sliced and seeds removed
2 onions, chopped
1 teaspoon each of paprika, cinnamon, cumin, and turmeric. Alternatively, you can use 1½ tablespoons of ras el hanout spice blend
1-2 teaspoons powdered ginger
½ teaspoon salt
½ teaspoon black pepper
8-12 green olives
Cilantro for garnish

1 Add all the ingredients except cilantro to a large saucepan and cover with water.

2 Bring to a boil and simmer for around 40 minutes or until the chicken is cooked and tender.

3 Once the meat is tender, remove the chicken from the pan, strip the meat, and add back into the tagine, discarding the skin and bones.

4 The tagine can be served alone or with Cauliflower Rice (page 154) topped with fresh cilantro.

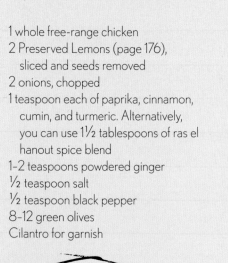
PREPARATION TIME: 15 minutes
COOKING TIME: 40 minutes
SERVES: 4-6

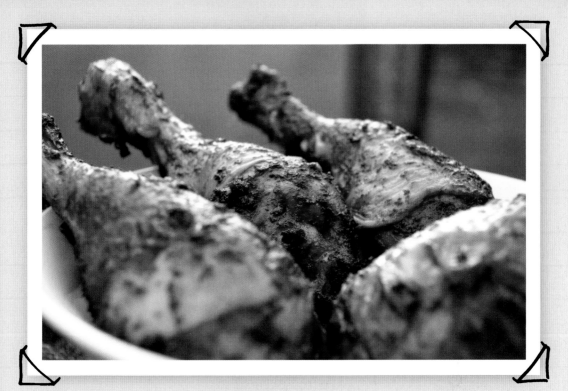

Sweet and Spicy Chicken

We like to make a large batch of these on the weekend, as they're always popular with friends and family. They are also great served cold as a snack or light lunch.

1 tablespoon olive oil or coconut oil
1 tablespoon honey
Juice of 1 lime
1 teaspoon allspice
½ teaspoon cinnamon
½ teaspoon cumin
1 teaspoon smoked paprika
1 teaspoon cayenne chili powder
1 teaspoon salt
1-inch piece of ginger, peeled and chopped
2 garlic cloves, finely chopped
   (or 1 teaspoon garlic powder)
12 chicken drumsticks

1 Preheat oven to 350°F.

2 Mix all the ingredients except for the chicken in a bowl. If using coconut oil, be sure to melt it first. Keep mixing until all the ingredients have blended together and formed a paste.

3 Now fully coat the chicken in the marinade and place on a baking sheet. Cook for 30-35 minutes.

PREPARATION TIME: 15 minutes
COOKING TIME: 30-35 minutes
SERVES: 4-5

Be sure not to drown the chicken in the marinade—otherwise, it won't get crispy.

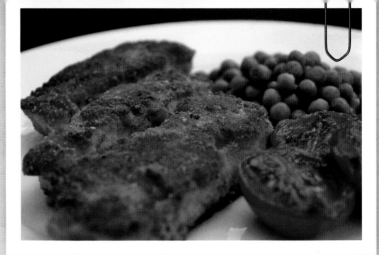

Fish Fingers

This is a great meal for kids and kids at heart ... just as good as the real thing. No one will ever know it's a healthy option in disguise.

2 5-ounce fillets of cod or haddock
1 egg
1 tablespoon almond flour (or finely
    ground almonds)
Salt and pepper to taste
½ teaspoon smoked paprika
½ teaspoon cayenne chili
1 tablespoon coconut oil, plus
    more for the pan

1 The day before you plan to eat the fish fingers, steam the fish for 10-15 minutes until cooked.

2 Remove from the steamer and place in a bowl. Mash the fish together and place on a baking sheet lined with parchment paper. (Ideally a rectangle-shaped sheet, 1 inch in height—about the height of a fish finger!) Cover and place in freezer overnight.

3 The next day, preheat oven to 350°F.

4 Beat the egg in a bowl. In a separate bowl, mix together the ground almonds, salt, pepper, smoked paprika, and cayenne chili. Grease a baking dish with a little oil.

5 Heat the coconut oil in a pan over low heat. While this is heating, remove the fish from the freezer and use a sharp knife to cut it into fish finger shapes.

PREPARATION TIME: 15-20 minutes
(Prepare the fish the day before)
COOKING TIME: 10-15 minutes
SERVES: 2

6 Coat each piece in the beaten egg and then roll in the ground almond mixture until fully coated. Place each fish finger in the pan to cook for 2-3 minutes on each side until crispy.

7 Transfer the fish fingers to the prepared baking sheet, and bake for 10-15 minutes until the coating is nice and golden.

Serve with
Fresh homemade Ketchup (page 172)

FISH, CHIPS, AND MUSHY PEAS

It wouldn't be a recipe book without this good ol' British favorite!

For the Chips
2 sweet potatoes, chopped
 into fries
1 tablespoon ghee or
 butter, melted
Salt and pepper to taste

For the Fish
1 egg
1 tablespoon almond
 flour (or finely ground
 almonds)
Salt and pepper to taste
1 tablespoon coconut oil
2 5-ounce haddock fillets

For the Mush Peas
1 cup frozen peas
1 tablespoon ghee or butter

1 Preheat oven to 350°F.

2 To prepare the chips, place the chopped sweet potatoes on a baking sheet and coat with 1 tablespoon melted ghee or butter, season with salt and pepper, and place in the oven.

3 Beat the egg in a bowl and set aside. Place the ground almonds in a separate bowl, add salt and pepper, and mix.

4 Heat the coconut oil in a saucepan over low heat. As this heats through, dip the fish fillets into the beaten egg and coat in the ground almond mixture.

5 Once the fish is coated nicely, place into the pan and cook for 2-3 minutes on each side to seal until golden and crispy. Repeat this with the second fillet.

6 After both have cooked for 2-3 minutes in the coconut oil, place them on a baking dish (add a little drop of the coconut oil to the dish and spread around to ensure the fillets don't stick to the pan).

7 Place the fish in the oven and cook for 10-15 minutes. While the fish and sweet potato chips are cooking, prepare the mushy peas.

8 Steam the frozen peas for 5 minutes until cooked through and soft. Place the peas in a bowl and add the remaining butter. Mash until creamy.

9 Once the fish and chips are cooked, serve and enjoy this healthy take on a traditional favorite.

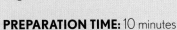

PREPARATION TIME: 10 minutes
COOKING TIME: 20-25 minutes
SERVES: 2

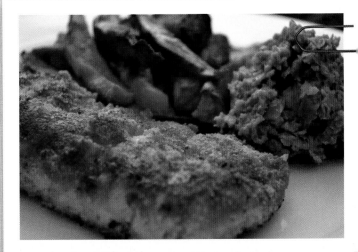

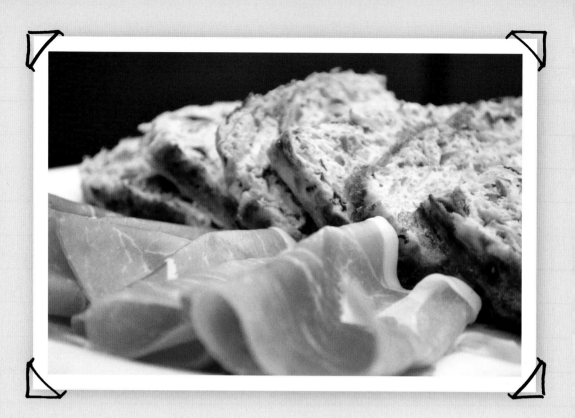

ROSEMARY LOAF

A Saturday afternoon favorite of ours after a long week. We love to serve this with a platter of cold meats, roasted nuts, olives, and a nice red wine.

Coconut oil to grease the loaf pan
10 eggs
Salt and pepper to taste
1 zucchini
1 tablespoon chopped fresh rosemary
5 Sun-Dried Tomatoes, chopped
   (page 168)

- - - - - - - - -

PREPARATION TIME: 10 minutes
COOKING TIME: 30 minutes
SERVES: 4

- - - - - - - -

1 Preheat oven to 350°F.

2 Grease a loaf pan with coconut oil or line it with parchment paper.

3 Place the eggs in a large mixing bowl and beat until the whites and yolks are blended. Season with salt and pepper.

4 Grate the zucchini into the beaten egg. Stir in the rosemary and sun-dried tomatoes.

5 Pour the mixture into the greased loaf pan and bake for 30 minutes. Use a knife to check it is cooked in the middle; the knife should come out clean if it is.

《 TIP 》

Adding 2-3 crushed garlic cloves before baking makes this a fantastic alternative to garlic bread.

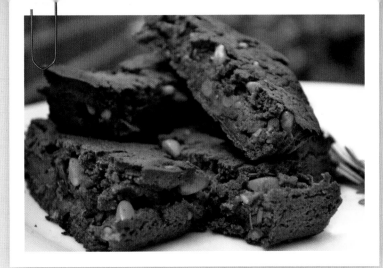

Chestnut Tea Cake

If you insist on indulging in some bread, one made with chestnut flour is a good choice. This particular recipe is Tuscan and traditionally enjoyed with a glass of dessert wine. However, we couldn't help but notice the combination of sweet chestnut flour, raisins, and crunchy pine nuts resembled the good old British tea cake, so we think it is best served with a lovely cup of tea!

1 cup chestnut flour
Warm water
3 tablespoons extra virgin olive oil, plus
    more for drizzling
2 tablespoons raisins (soaked in
    warm water for 10 minutes)
2 tablespoons pine nuts
1 tablespoon fresh rosemary
Pinch of salt

1 Preheat oven to 350°F.

2 Sift the flour and salt into a bowl and add enough warm water to make a liquid batter. You may wish to use a whisk to prevent lumps from forming, but it isn't essential.

3 Add 3 tablespoons of olive oil and the raisins (you must soak these as it really makes a difference to the sweetness and texture).

4 Mix the batter and pour into a 12-inch cake pan lined with parchment paper.

5 Sprinkle the pine nuts and rosemary on top of the batter and drizzle with a little more olive oil.

6 Bake for about 1 hour until it is dark and crispy on top but moist in the middle.

7 Serve warm with a large pot of tea (green if possible).

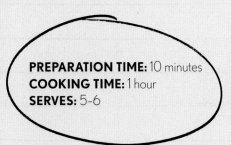

PREPARATION TIME: 10 minutes
COOKING TIME: 1 hour
SERVES: 5-6

Cauliflower Pizza

Pizza in a healthy recipe book ... surely not! Relax, we've made it healthy, using grated cauliflower as the secret ingredient in our yummy grain-free crust. Feel free to experiment with different toppings, including fish, meats, hard-boiled eggs, veggies, and olives. We included cheese in our version, as a pizza without cheese just wouldn't be taken seriously.

For the Crust
1 medium cauliflower, grated
2 eggs
1 8-ounce ball of buffalo mozzarella
Salt and pepper to taste
½ teaspoon garlic powder

For the Sauce
2 tablespoons olive oil
4 medium tomatoes, chopped
2-3 garlic cloves, crushed or
    finely chopped
Handful of fresh basil, chopped
Salt and pepper to taste

Topping Ideas
½ ball of buffalo mozzarella
    (around 4 ounces), sliced
4 ounces goat cheese
¼ green pepper, sliced
½ red pepper, sliced
3-4 chestnut mushrooms, sliced
4-5 slices pepperoni
5 black olives, sliced (We do green,
    something popular with us Brits.)

Serve with
A crisp green salad and a good movie

- - - - - - - -

PREPARATION TIME:
15-20 minutes
COOKING TIME:
45-50 minutes
SERVES: 4-6

- - - - - - - -

1 Preheat oven to 350°F.

2 Grate the cauliflower and place in the steamer for about 4-5 minutes to soften. Leave to cool slightly.

3 Beat the eggs and finely chop the mozzarella. In a blender, mix the mozzarella, cauliflower, eggs, and seasonings at medium speed until a dough-like paste forms.

4 Top a baking sheet with parchment paper and add a little olive oil to prevent sticking. Add the pizza dough to the tray and spread out to make a circle. The base should be around ⅓-inch thick.

5 Place in the oven and bake for about 30-35 minutes, until golden around the edges.

6 While the base is cooking, start to make the sauce and prepare the toppings.

7 Heat some olive oil in a pan and stir in the tomatoes, garlic, basil, salt, and pepper. Cook over low heat, stirring occasionally.

8 While the sauce is heating through, make sure all your toppings are chopped and ready to be placed on the pizza. Once the sauce is cooked through, spin through the blender just long enough to beat out the tomato skins.

9 When your base is looking nice and golden, it's time to top your pizza. Remove the base from the oven and add the tomato sauce and your toppings.

10 Place the pizza back in the oven and bake for 10-15 minutes until the cheese is melted.

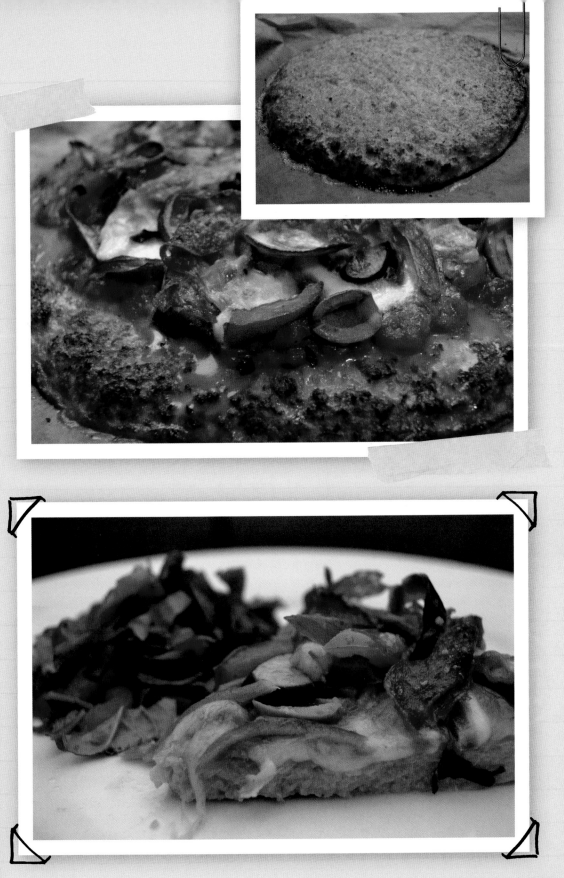

Slow-Cooked Anchovy Lamb

Our butcher suggested we try a lamb shoulder joint for a change one Sunday. We slow-cooked the joint for 3–4 hours in anchovy butter—words cannot describe how good this tastes!

For the Lamb

3 pounds lamb shoulder
3 tablespoons butter, softened (or substitute goose fat, beef fat, or lard for a dairy-free option)
Leaves of 3–4 rosemary sprigs, chopped
4 garlic cloves, finely chopped
Juice of half a lemon
8–10 anchovy fillets or 3 teaspoons anchovy paste
1 tablespoon mustard seeds

For the Sides

2 sweet potatoes, peeled and chopped into cubes
1 tablespoon butter or olive oil
Salt and pepper to taste
Head of broccoli, cut into bite-size florets

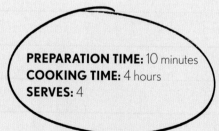

PREPARATION TIME: 10 minutes
COOKING TIME: 4 hours
SERVES: 4

1 Preheat oven to 300°F.

2 With a sharp knife, score several shallow criss-crosses across the fatty side of the lamb.

3 Combine the butter, rosemary, garlic, lemon juice, anchovies, and mustard seeds in a bowl, and spread mixture evenly over the lamb joint.

4 Cook for 4 hours. You may need to cover the lamb with aluminum foil partway through to keep it from crisping too much. You know it's cooked when you can pull the meat apart easily with two forks.

5 Remove the lamb from the oven, and lift out of the roasting tray. Cover with foil, place a tea towel on top, and leave it to rest. Scoop out most of the lamb fat (set aside in a jar for cooking another meal), leaving the meat juices in the roasting tray to be used as gravy.

6 Steam sweet potato for about 15 minutes or so. Once cooked, remove from steamer and add broccoli.

7 While broccoli steams for 8 minutes or so, mash the sweet potato with butter or olive oil, then season with salt and pepper. Slice the lamb and serve with the steamed broccoli and mashed sweet potatoes.

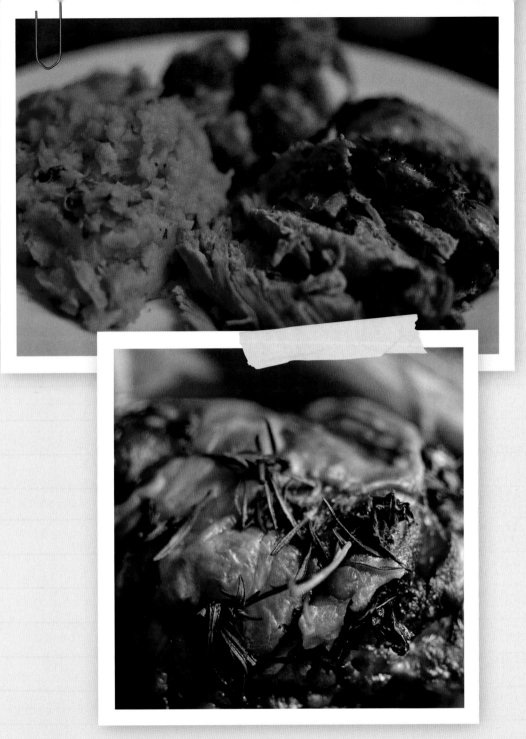

SIDES

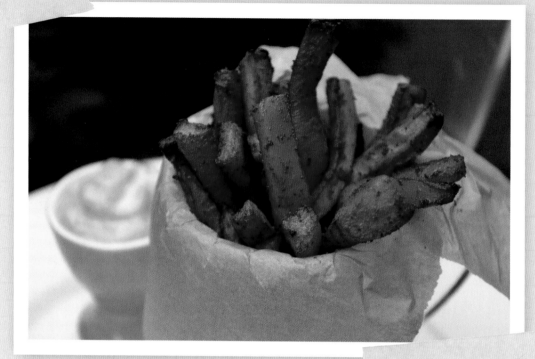

SPICY CARROT FRIES

A fantastic side, snack, or starter. Delicious with Homemade Mayonnaise (page 173).

6 large carrots
½ teaspoon chili powder
2–3 garlic cloves, finely chopped
2 tablespoons oil (macadamia,
  olive, butter, ghee, or goose fat)
Salt and pepper to taste

1 Preheat oven to 325°F.

2 Slice the carrots into french fry-size sticks.

3 In a bowl, mix together chili, garlic, and oil.

4 Toss carrots in the mixture and spread out flat on a baking sheet.

5 Bake for 20–30 minutes until cooked to your liking.

6 Just before serving, season to taste with salt and pepper.

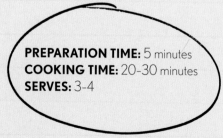

PREPARATION TIME: 5 minutes
COOKING TIME: 20–30 minutes
SERVES: 3–4

CELERIAC FRIES

Not many people use celeriac in their weekly cooking adventures, often because they are unsure of how to cook the root vegetable. It's great cooked and mashed or added to savory soups and stews ... and it's packed with loads of micronutrients! This recipe works well with sweet potatoes, parsnips, and carrots, too!

2 tablespoons goose fat, beef fat, coconut oil, or ghee for cooking
1 tablespoon chopped fresh rosemary or mixed herbs
2 garlic cloves, finely chopped
1 celeriac, peeled and cut into fries (You can also use sweet potatoes, parsnips, or carrots)

PREPARATION TIME: 10 minutes
COOKING TIME: 1 hour
SERVES: 3-4

1 Preheat oven to 325°F.

2 Melt the fat (you can melt it in a small baking dish while the oven is preheating).

3 Once the fat is melted, stir in the rosemary and garlic.

4 Grease a large baking sheet or line it with parchment paper.

5 Scatter the fries across the baking sheet, and use your hands to toss the fries in the rosemary-garlic oil.

6 Place in the oven. These usually take about an hour to crisp up on low heat. After the first 30 minutes, stir and toss the fries again to re-coat in the fat. Once the fries are cooked to your liking, remove from the oven and cool.

Great with the Tarragon Roast Chicken and Chestnut Stuffing (page 139)

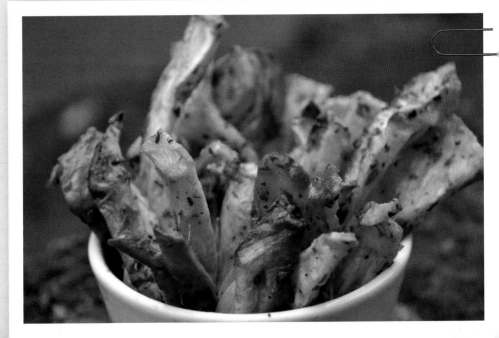

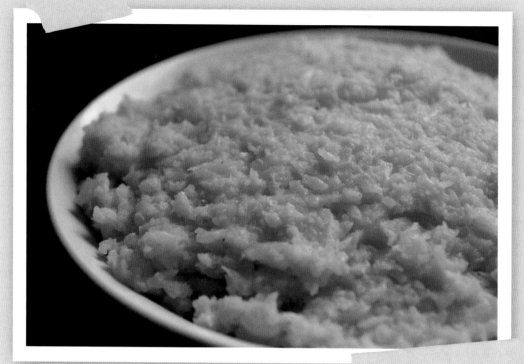

CAULIFLOWER RICE

Grains like rice and couscous just cannot compete with this nutritional superfood, so turn your cauliflower into rice and no one will ever know the difference.

1 tablespoon butter, ghee, or olive oil
1 large cauliflower, grated
A splash of cream (optional)
Chives, chopped (optional)
Salt and pepper to taste

1 In a large saucepan, heat the oil or fat over low heat.

2 Add the cauliflower, cream, and chives (if desired) to the pan and stir-fry.

3 Stir consistently to stop the cauliflower from burning.

4 After 5 minutes, taste to check the consistency and serve as soon as it's soft enough.

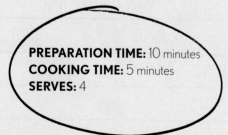

PREPARATION TIME: 10 minutes
COOKING TIME: 5 minutes
SERVES: 4

TIP

Be adventurous and experiment with flavorful additions like herbs, spices, onions, scallions, garlic, or mushrooms.

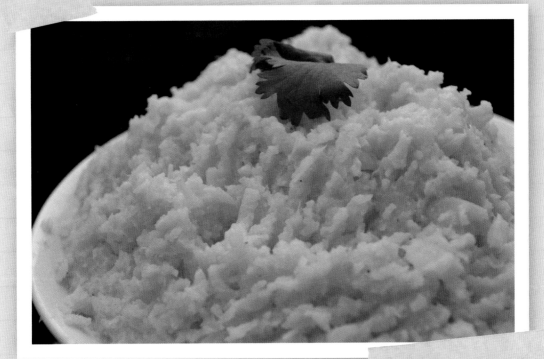

Cauliflower Mash

Even if you aren't the biggest fan of cauliflower, we bet you'll still love this awesome creamy mash. It's the perfect low-carbohydrate topping for Primal Shepherd's Pie (page 131). You can also try adding other herbs, onion, garlic, or spices to create your own must-have mash.

1 large cauliflower, grated
1 tablespoon butter, ghee, or olive oil
1-2 tablespoons heavy cream
Salt and pepper to taste

1 Steam the cauliflower it is until soft, about 4-5 minutes.

2 Place in a large bowl, add the fat and cream, and season to taste with salt and pepper.

3 Mash until the mixture is a smooth, creamy consistency.

PREPARATION TIME: 10 minutes
COOKING TIME: 8 minutes
SERVES: 4-6

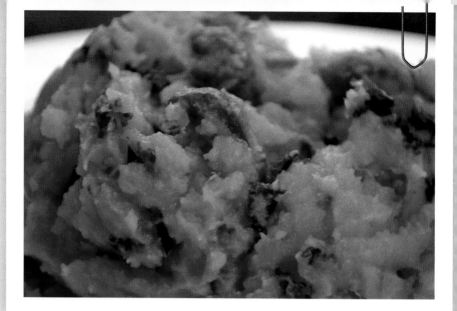

Kale and Chorizo Mash

Kale is one of the most nutrient-dense vegetables on the planet. When you add it to chorizo and mashed sweet potatoes, it turns into a truly epic side dish.

2 sweet potatoes, chopped
3 kale leaves, chopped
2 small chorizo sausages, chopped
1 tablespoon extra virgin olive oil
Salt and pepper to taste

PREPARATION TIME: 10 minutes
COOKING TIME: 25 minutes
SERVES: 2

1 Place the sweet potato in a steamer and cook for 10 minutes. Leave enough room to add the kale.

2 Add the kale to the steamer and cook for 5 minutes.

3 While the vegetables are steaming, panfry the chorizo over low heat.

4 Once the potato and kale are cooked, remove from the steamer.

5 Mash the potato with a fork or vegetable masher and add the olive oil.

6 Mix in the chopped kale and the cooked chorizo. Season to taste with salt and pepper.

Butternut Smash

This way of preparing butternut squash takes out the hassle of peeling and chopping. Once you've baked the squash, just scoop out the softened flesh and you've got instant mash!

1 butternut squash, sliced in half
Salt and pepper

PREPARATION TIME: 2 minutes
COOKING TIME: 25-30 minutes
SERVES: 6

1 Preheat oven to 350°F.

2 Scoop the seeds out of each squash half and discard them.

3 Place the squash on a baking sheet and bake for 25-30 minutes.

4 Once cooked (the flesh should be soft enough that you can easily insert a knife), use a fork to scrape out the flesh and place in a serving bowl.

 It's easiest to cook a half or a whole squash at one time. Save any leftovers for adding to soups and stews.

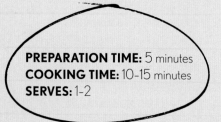

BUBBLE AND SQUEAK

A hearty dish of fried leftover vegetables makes a great side or a small meal. This traditional British favorite is ideally made with butternut squash or sweet potato for extra substance, but any leftover veggies will do.

Ghee or coconut oil for the pan
Leftover vegetables from your Sunday roast (such as sweet potatoes, broccoli, carrots, zucchini, celery)

1 Mash together the leftover vegetables from a previously cooked dinner.

2 Heat the oil in a pan over low heat and then add the bubble and squeak. Keep mixing until all the vegetables are heated through.

3 Serve on its own or with the leftover meat from your Sunday roast.

PREPARATION TIME: 5 minutes
COOKING TIME: 10-15 minutes
SERVES: 1-2

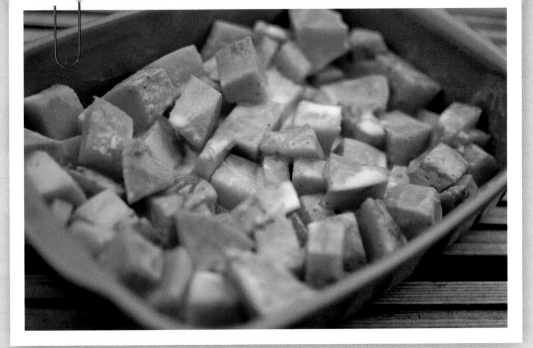

CINNAMON COCONUT SQUASH

A sweet vegetable side dish that can also pull duty as a great stand-alone snack.

Half a butternut squash
4 ounces coconut milk
1 garlic clove, finely chopped
½ teaspoon cinnamon
Salt and pepper to taste

1 Preheat oven to 350°F.

2 Chop the butternut squash into cubes and place in a small baking dish.

3 Pour the coconut milk over the squash, sprinkle with garlic and cinnamon, and stir to coat.

4 Bake for 35-40 minutes.

5 Just before serving, season with a little salt and pepper.

PREPARATION TIME: 5 minutes
COOKING TIME: 35-40 minutes
SERVES: 2

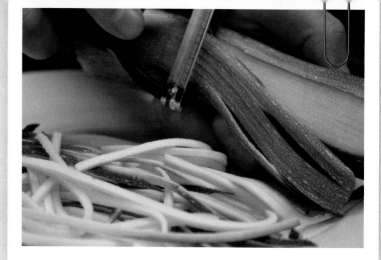

Vegetable Spaghetti

A healthy substitute to pasta! If you don't already own a julienne peeler, get one. It's an absolute must for quick, easy vegetable spaghetti.

Vegetable of your choice: carrots, zucchini, butternut squash

1 Use a julienne peeler to slice the vegetables into spaghetti-like strips.

2 The strips can either be cooked in a steamer or gently sautéed in a little oil in a frying pan until the vegetables have softened.

PREPARATION TIME: 5 minutes
COOKING TIME: 15 minutes

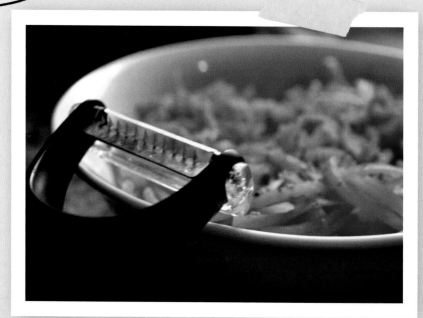

Vegetable Kebabs

This is a simple vegetable side dish that can add some Mediterranean flavor to any fish or meat dish.

1 red pepper
1 yellow pepper
1 white onion
2 zucchinis
1 tablespoon ghee, olive oil, or butter
1 tablespoon mixed herbs
Salt and pepper to taste
6-8 fresh rosemary sprigs or
   kebab sticks

1 Preheat oven to 350°F.

2 Chop all the vegetables into large chunks.

3 Melt the fat and add the mixed herbs, salt, and pepper. Coat the vegetables with the mixture.

4 Thread the vegetables onto the kebab sticks or rosemary sprigs. Remember, if using rosemary sprigs, be sure to skewer vegetables at the bottom of the stalk.

5 Place the kebabs on a baking sheet and bake for 20 minutes, turning occasionally.

PREPARATION TIME: 10 minutes
COOKING TIME: 20 minutes
SERVES: 3-4

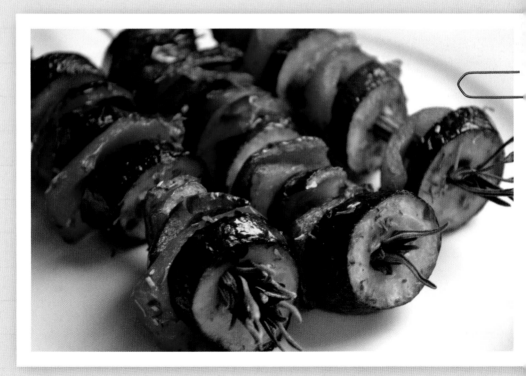

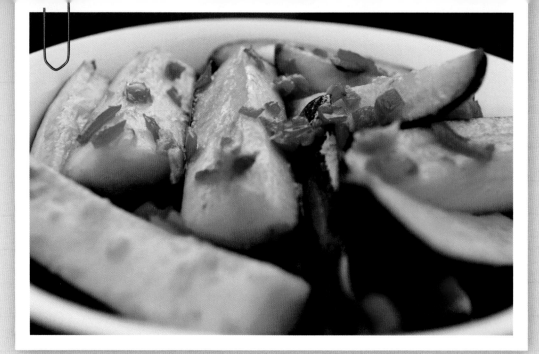

Chunky Zucchini Fries

This tasty side serving of vegetables can accompany anything and takes virtually no time to put together. Cutting the zucchini into chunky fries makes this a really hearty side.

3 large zucchinis
Coconut oil for the pan
1 garlic clove, finely chopped
½ teaspoon chili flakes (optional)
Salt and pepper to taste

PREPARATION TIME: 5 minutes
COOKING TIME: 8 minutes
SERVES: 2

1 Chop the zucchini into chunky fries (no need to peel them first).

2 Melt the oil in a pan over low heat, and add the garlic and zucchini.

3 Sprinkle with the chili flakes.

4 Sauté to your liking. (It's best to keep checking by crunching on a fry every now and then.)

5 Just before serving, season with a little salt and pepper.

Lemon and Thyme Baked Carrots

Carrots are often just served up as a steamed side. Here, we've cooked them in citrus juices with garlic and herbs. Give it a go—you'll never serve plain carrots again.

2-4 large carrots
Juice of half a lemon
1 garlic clove, finely chopped
1 tablespoon fresh thyme
Salt and pepper to taste

1 Preheat oven to 350°F.

2 Slice the carrots and place in a small baking dish.

3 Squeeze lemon juice over the carrots and sprinkle with garlic and thyme.

4 Bake for 25-30 minutes or until the carrots are cooked to your liking. Season to taste with salt and pepper.

PREPARATION TIME: 5 minutes
COOKING TIME: 25-30 minutes
SERVES: 2

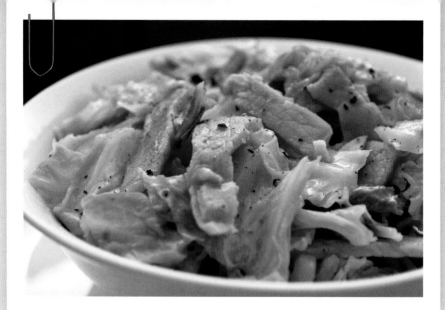

BUTTERED SAVOY CABBAGE (WITH OR WITHOUT BACON!)

Cabbage is delicious cooked in butter, and you can top it with bacon for a tasty treat.

1 whole Savoy cabbage, sliced
1 tablespoon or so of butter or ghee
Salt and pepper to taste
2-3 slices of uncooked bacon
   (optional)

PREPARATION TIME: 2 minutes
COOKING TIME: 8-10 minutes
SERVES: 4

1 Melt the butter or ghee in a pan over a low heat.

2 Place the cabbage in the pan, adding the bacon if desired.

3 Mix well and gently stir-fry for 6-8 minutes. Season to taste with salt and pepper.

4 Once the cabbage is cooked to your liking, place in a serving bowl. Feel free to add more butter.

SPINACH, SUN-DRIED TOMATOES, AND PINE NUTS

Sun-dried tomatoes with olive oil and toasted pine nuts make a simple addition to sautéed spinach.

1 tablespoon pine nuts
Water
3 large handfuls or so of spinach
2 or 3 Sun-Dried Tomatoes
   (page 168), chopped
Salt and pepper to taste

1 Place a non-stick pan over low heat.

2 Add the pine nuts to the pan and gently stir-fry (no fats or oil needed). Keep moving the pine nuts around the pan to ensure they cook evenly and do not burn. Once they are toasted, remove from the pan and set aside.

3 Add a little water to the pan and add the spinach.

4 Gently stir-fry for 2–3 minutes, until the spinach has wilted.

5 Once the spinach is cooked to your liking, place in a serving bowl and drizzle with olive oil.

6 Top with the sun-dried tomatoes and toasted pine nuts.

7 Season to taste with salt and pepper and serve.

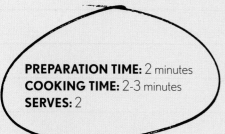

PREPARATION TIME: 2 minutes
COOKING TIME: 2-3 minutes
SERVES: 2

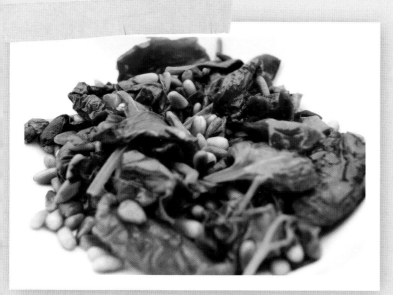

HOW TO PIMP A SALAD

HOW TO PIMP A SALAD

When it comes to salads, many people envision a large plate of leaves—hardly anything to get excited about. But we treat salads like every other meal and infuse them with lots of intense flavors. Here are a few simple ways to pimp your salad.

ROASTED PEPPERS

These add sweetness, texture, and Mediterranean flavors to your leafy greens.

1 red pepper
1 yellow pepper
1 green pepper
1 tablespoon extra virgin olive oil

1 Preheat oven to 300°F.

2 Slice peppers into quarters and discard the core and the seeds.

3 Lightly bake the peppers for 30-40 minutes until soft. Dress with olive oil and toss with salad leaves.

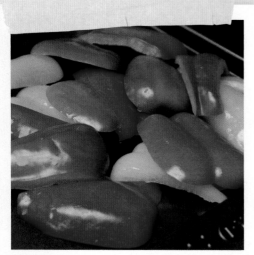

《TIP》 We cook plenty of peppers and store them in a glass jar with extra virgin olive oil and a teaspoon of mixed herbs and chopped garlic.

Soaked Sun-Dried Tomatoes

We know you can buy these in nearly every supermarket, but they are often preserved in poor quality oil. Soaking your own ensures maximum quality and taste. Here's how: start with organic dried tomatoes sold in a bag.

1 Soak the dried tomatoes in purified water overnight to soften. Drain the water and place the plumped tomatoes in a glass jar.

2 Cover with good quality extra virgin olive oil. You can infuse the oil with garlic or fresh herbs like rosemary, thyme, or basil. Store in the refrigerator.

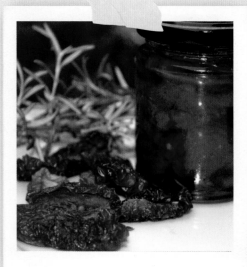

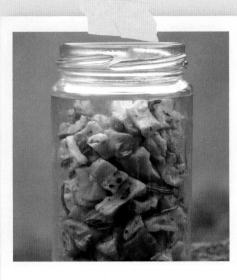

Root Vegetable Croutons

A great way to add some substance to a salad and boost vital antioxidants. Our favorites are celeriac, parsnip, or crispy sweet potato croutons.

Root vegetables (sweet potatoes, celeriac, parsnips, or carrots)
2 tablespoons of fat for cooking (goose fat or beef fat from your Sunday roast, or you can use coconut oil or ghee)
1 tablespoon fresh or dried herbs (rosemary and thyme, or mixed herbs work well)
2 garlic cloves, crushed (optional)

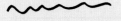

PREPARATION TIME: 10 minutes
COOKING TIME: 1 hour

1 Preheat oven to 300°F. Peel and dice the vegetables. Melt the fat (you can place it in a ramekin or other small baking dish to melt in the oven while it's warming). Once the fat is melted, stir in the herbs and crushed garlic.

2 Grease a large baking sheet or line it with parchment paper. Scatter the diced vegetables across the baking sheet and coat with the melted fat, herbs, and garlic. Use your (clean!) hands to toss the croutons in the fat and make sure all of them are coated.

3 Place in the oven. After 30 minutes, stir or toss the croutons again to coat in the fat. Once the vegetables are crispy to your liking (they usually take an hour to crisp up on low heat), remove from the oven and cool.

Toasted Walnuts

One of the healthiest ways to prepare nuts is to soak them in water with a pinch of salt overnight, and then slowly roast them in the oven on low heat, around 100 degrees, for 3-4 hours. This breaks down many of the digestive irritants in the nuts but also enhances the flavor and crunchy texture, making them the perfect salad topping. Store the nuts in an airtight glass jar.

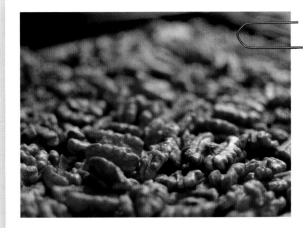

Dips and condiments

Ketchup

We used to be huge ketchup fans, but decided to cut it out due to the high sugar content. But there are still occasions when we get the urge, so here's a sugar-free version of our favorite condiment. We tried and tested many paleo ketchup recipes, and this was easily the best, created by Sébastien Noël of PaleoDietLifestyle.com.

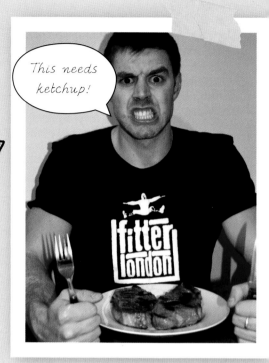

2 6-ounce cans tomato paste
2 tablespoons apple cider vinegar or lemon juice
¼ teaspoon dry mustard powder
3 ounces water
¼ teaspoon cinnamon
¼ teaspoon salt
A dash of ground cloves
A dash of ground allspice
A dash cayenne pepper (optional)

Combine all the ingredients in a bowl and whisk well to combine. Refrigerate overnight to let the flavors develop, and enjoy!

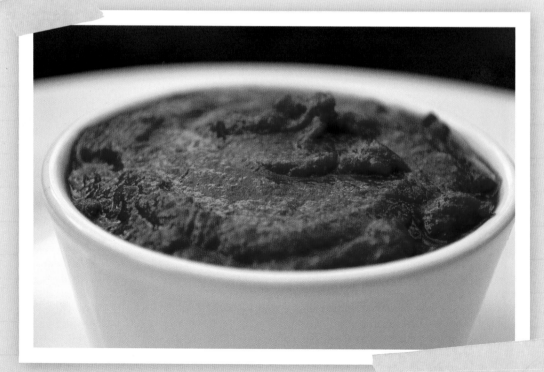

Homemade Mayonnaise

When you make mayonnaise yourself, it's actually an incredibly healthy dressing for salads and dishes, and it goes great with Spicy Carrot Fries (page 152). Many commercial mayonnaises tend to use cheap, poor quality oils and contain additives and preservatives to increase the shelf life. A basic mayonnaise recipe calls for 1 cup of oil. Using just olive oil can dominate the mayonnaise, so it's best to combine the oils.

2 egg yolks
3 teaspoons lemon juice
1 cup oil

Oil Options
Our favorite blend is 3 parts macadamia oil to 1 part avocado oil, but experiment with any of the following.

* Olive oil
* Avocado oil
* Macadamia oil
* Coconut oil (melt beforehand)

1 Put the yolks in a blender or food processor with the lemon juice and mix together.

2 Start the mixer and **very slowly** add the oil. Start by doing this drop by drop to ensure the mixture emulsifies. If you add the oil too quickly, this won't happen and there's no going back!

3 As you add the oil, the mixture will emulsify and thicken into a mayonnaise texture. Once this happens, you can add the oil at a quicker pace.

4 Once all the oil is added, keep mixing and tasting until you are happy with the final mayonnaise.

5 Store in a glass jar in the fridge.

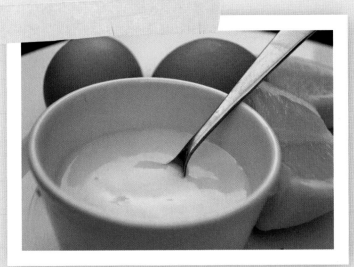

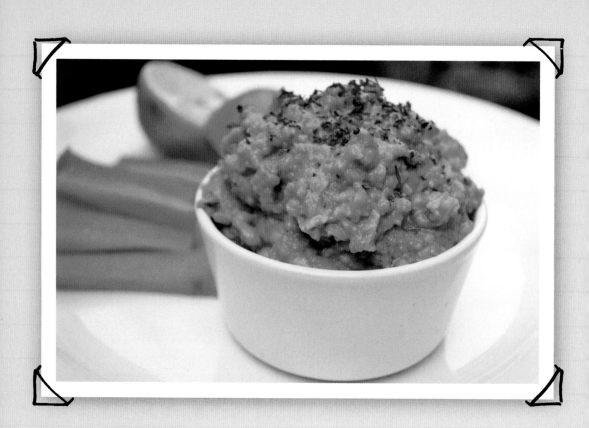

Guacamole

This guacamole doesn't last long, and for good reason—it doesn't have any of the preservatives you often find in store-bought varieties. It's so quick to prepare, and there's rarely any left over when we make it.

2 medium avocados
1 tomato, finely chopped
¼ cup finely chopped fresh cilantro
Juice of half a lemon or 1 whole lime
Salt and pepper to taste
½ red onion, finely chopped (optional)

1 Slice the avocados in half and scoop out the flesh. Mash the flesh in a bowl with a fork until it forms a creamy consistency.

2 Stir in the other ingredients and taste. Add more herbs, seasoning, or lemon juice until it hits the spot.

3 Eat this right away or store in the refrigerator.

Oil Infusions

Infuse the oils you use for dressings with lots of fresh or dried herbs and spices to boost flavors and antioxidants, and to increase the anti-inflammatory effect of your food. Place your oil in a glass jar (jam jar or similar). If using fresh herbs, bruise them a little first (rub or crush the leaves to release the oils), or just add dried herbs. Place a lid on the jar and keep it in a cool, dark space to infuse for a week. Taste the oil, and if it needs more flavor, let it steep longer or add more herbs and spices. Explore different combinations! The following work well.

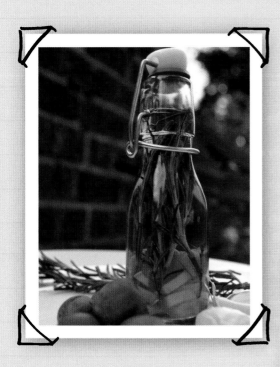

- Garlic and rosemary
- Basil and sun-dried tomato
- Lemon zest and chili
- Rosemary and thyme

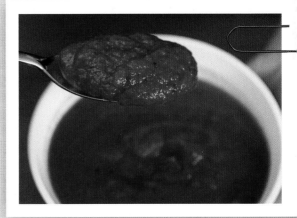

QUICK & EASY TOMATO SAUCE

2 tablespoons olive oil
4 medium tomatoes, chopped
2-3 garlic cloves, finely chopped
1 teaspoon thyme
Salt and pepper to taste

1 Heat the olive oil in a pan and stir in the tomatoes, garlic, thyme, salt, and pepper. Cook over low heat, stirring occasionally.

2 Once the sauce is cooked through, spin through the blender just long enough to beat out the tomato skins.

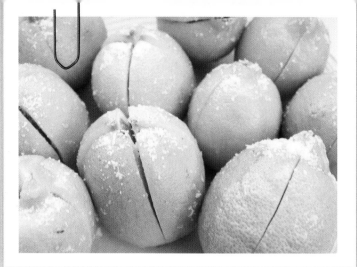

6 to 8 lemons
½ cup or so of kosher salt

EQUIPMENT
One 6-cup canning jar with
a tight-fitting lid

1 Sterilize jar in boiling water and wash the lemons.

2 Sprinkle 1 tablespoon of salt on the bottom of the jar.

3 Cut the lemons into quarters without cutting all the way through to the bottom. The lemons should open up but remain attached at the base.

4 Sprinkle about a tablespoon of salt into each cut lemon, and pack tightly into the jar (really cram them in), sprinkling a coating of salt over each layer as you go. Add additional flavorings and put the lid on the jar..

5 The lemons will release some juice as you pack them in, and even more over the next two days. Make sure that by day two the lemons are completely covered with juice. If you need to, squeeze fresh lemon juice it into the jar.

6 Let the lemons sit at room temperature for at least two weeks, ideally thirty days. Shake the jar periodically to distribute the salt and juice.

7 After thirty days or so, remove the lemons from the liquid and rinse well to remove the salt. Scrape out the pulp from each lemon and slice.

8 Cover the slices with olive oil and put them in the refrigerator, where they'll keep for at least 6 months.

PRESERVED LEMONS

Preserved lemons lend Moroccan dishes their intense flavor. Add thin strips to braised lamb near the end of the cooking process for a brighter flavor. Or finely chop a strip with a shallot and parsley, and mash in some olive oil or butter to use as a spread on top of seafood or chicken. Also great added to roasted vegetables, sprinkled into salads, or diced and mixed with olives for an appetizer. This recipe comes to us courtesy of Mark's Daily Apple.

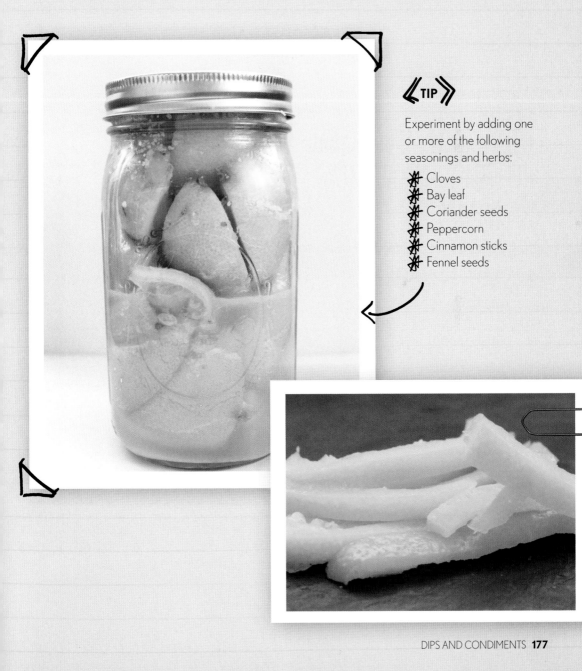

《 TIP 》

Experiment by adding one or more of the following seasonings and herbs:

- Cloves
- Bay leaf
- Coriander seeds
- Peppercorn
- Cinnamon sticks
- Fennel seeds

HEALTHY SNACKS

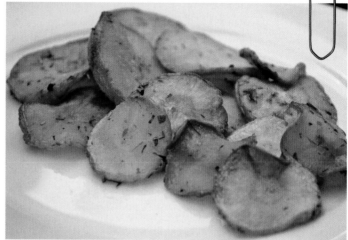

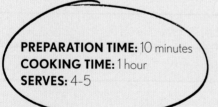

HOMEMADE KETTLE CHIPS

Chips made from root vegetables make a great substitute for potato chips. They taste so much better homemade, and that way you can ensure good quality fats are used. Experiment with different flavors like garlic, apple cider vinegar, salt, or chili. We use parsnips in this recipe, but beetroot, celeriac, and sweet potatoes also work well.

1 tablespoon of fat (goose
   fat or beef fat is best, or you can use
   coconut oil or ghee)
1 tablespoon fresh or dried herbs.
   (Rosemary and thyme or mixed
   herbs work well)
2 garlic cloves, finely chopped (optional)
2-3 parsnips, peeled and thinly sliced

PREPARATION TIME: 10 minutes
COOKING TIME: 1 hour
SERVES: 4-5

1 Preheat oven to 300°F.

2 Melt the fat (you can melt it in a small baking dish while the oven is preheating).

3 Once the fat is melted, stir in the herbs and garlic.

4 Grease a large baking sheet or line it with parchment paper.

5 Scatter the sliced parsnips across the sheet and coat them with the melted fat, herbs, and garlic. Use your clean hands to toss the chips in the fat and make sure all are coated.

6 Place the parsnips in the oven. These usually take an hour to crisp up on low heat. After the first 30 minutes, stir and toss the chips again to coat in the fat.

7 Once the parsnips are crispy to your liking, remove from the oven and cool. Best eaten straight away.

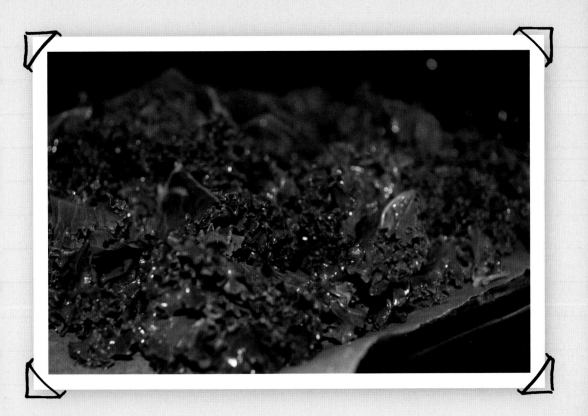

SALT AND VINEGAR KALE CHIPS

A great snack and a much healthier option than a bag of chips. Again, you can explore flavors with kale chips using garlic, mustard powder, and other spices.

6-8 kale leaves
2 tablespoons olive oil
1 teaspoon apple cider vinegar
¼ teaspoon salt

PREPARATION TIME: 10 minutes
COOKING TIME: 10 minutes
SERVES: 4-5

1 Preheat oven to 325°F.

2 Wash the kale and dry using a kitchen towel. Tear the leaves into small pieces.

3 Place the kale in a large bowl with the olive oil and apple cider vinegar. Toss in the oil and rub the leaves to make sure each is coated well.

4 Place on a baking sheet lined with parchment paper. Sprinkle with salt to taste.

5 Bake for 5 minutes, then turn the kale pieces to ensure they cook evenly. Bake for another 6-9 minutes.

6 Keep checking—smaller pieces cook quicker and may need to be removed from heat sooner.

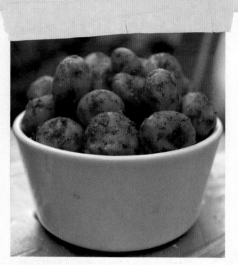

CHILI-ROASTED MACADAMIAS

We love macadamias. Not only are they the tastiest nuts going, they are also a good source of healthy, monounsaturated fats. Making your own versions of flavored nuts is always tastier and healthier—and it's so simple! Keep these in a glass jar as a healthy snack.

PREPARATION TIME: 2-3 minutes
COOKING TIME: 1 hour
SERVES: 8

8 ounces whole macadamia nuts
1 tablespoon olive oil
½ teaspoon salt
1 teaspoon curry powder
1 teaspoon ground cumin
1 teaspoon ground coriander
1 teaspoon chili powder

1 Preheat oven to 300°F. Line a baking sheet with parchment paper.

2 Place the nuts in a bowl and toss with the oil until well coated. Add the salt and spices, mixing well to coat the nuts evenly.

3 Spread the nuts over the prepared baking sheet.

4 Bake for 1 hour on low heat until the nuts are lightly browned. Remove from oven and allow to cool before serving.

Movie Mix

Our alternative to a bucket of popcorn, nachos, or ice cream when we go to the movies.

3 ounces dried mango
3.5-ounce 85 percent dark chocolate bar
3 ounces organic coconut flakes
7 ounces macadamia nuts

1 Break chocolate into squares. Use kitchen shears to cut the mango into small pieces.

2 Simply mix up all the ingredients into a trail mix. Place in a large glass jar, and when it's movie time, take a small serving with you.

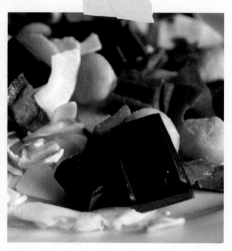

PREPARATION TIME: 5 minutes
COOKING TIME: N/A
SERVES: 4-5

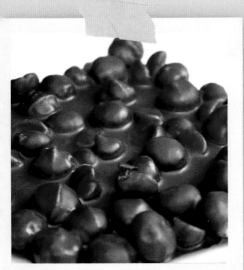

PREPARATION TIME: 10 minutes
COOKING TIME: 1 hour (if baking the nuts)
SERVES: 4

½ cup whole macadamias nuts (the bigger the better)
3.5-ounce 85 percent dark chocolate bar

 TIP This tastes best if the nuts are gently dry roasted in the oven, but you can skip this step and go straight to step 2.

Chocolate Macadamias

A Primal take on an American classic: M&M's—but without the sugary candy shell. We've replaced the peanuts with omega-3-rich macadamia nuts and married them with antioxidant-rich dark chocolate. Toasting the nuts adds to the flavor and texture.

1 Preheat oven to 300°F and line a baking sheet with parchment paper. Spread the nuts over the prepared baking sheet, and bake for 1 hour on low heat until the nuts are lightly browned.

2 To melt the chocolate, place a heat-proof glass bowl over a pan of boiling water to create a double boiler effect. Break chocolate into squares and place in the bowl to melt. Once the chocolate has melted to a liquid consistency, remove from the heat.

3 Add the macadamias to the chocolate. Pour onto a plate lined with a sheet of parchment paper.

4 Place in the fridge. Once the mixture has set (which usually takes 30 minutes), break into chunks. Store in a glass jar.

Toasted Coconut

Just one awesome ingredient:
½ cup coconut flakes

1 Preheat oven to 300°F and line a baking sheet with parchment paper. Spread the coconut flakes over the baking sheet so they can be cooked evenly.

2 Bake for 20 minutes or until the coconut is lightly browned. Store in a glass jar.

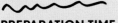

PREPARATION TIME: 2 minutes
COOKING TIME: 20 minutes
SERVES: 4

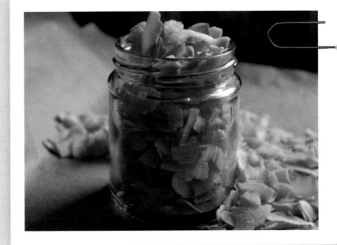

Cheats of Champions

! **WARNING**
These treats (although healthier)
should only be eaten **VERY**
occasionally!

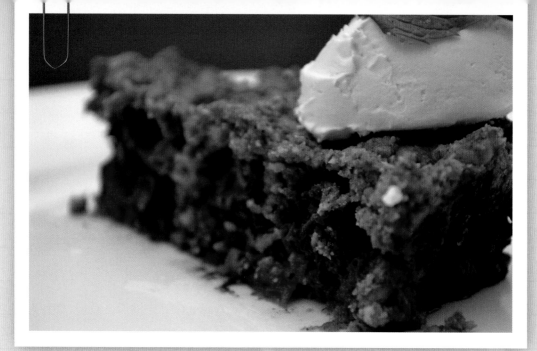

BLACKBERRY APPLE CRUMBLE

One of the best British fruit combos—all we did was add a crunchy nut topping. A great finish to your Sunday roast.

4 apples
1 pint fresh blackberries
1 cup ground almonds
2 tablespoons butter
1 cup coconut flakes
1 tablespoon raw honey or 2 teaspoons
    coconut sugar (optional)
1 tablespoon cinnamon
¾ cup chopped walnuts

Serve with
Whipped heavy cream (optional)

PREPARATION TIME: 10 minutes
COOKING TIME: 30-40 minutes
SERVES: 6

1 Preheat oven to 350°F.

2 Slice the apples and remove the cores.

3 Layer the apples and blackberries in a loaf pan.

4 Place the ground almonds and coconut in a bowl with the butter, honey, and cinnamon.

5 Using your hands, rub the fat into the ground almonds and coconut until the mixture has the consistency of breadcrumbs. Add the chopped walnuts and stir together with a spoon.

6 Place the crumble mixture on top of the fruit. There should be a ½-inch layer. If there are any gaps, simply sprinkle with some extra desiccated coconut.

7 Bake for 30-40 minutes until the crumble topping is golden brown and the fruit is soft.

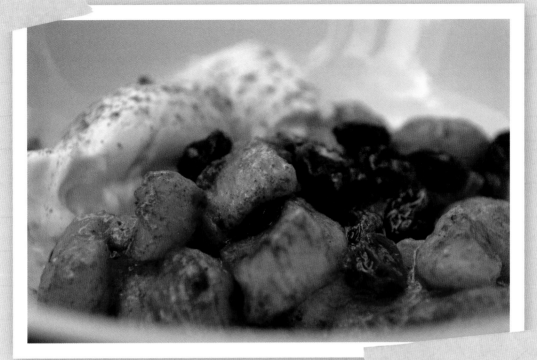

BREADLESS BUTTER PUDDING

A healthy version of the classic bread and butter pudding. We swapped out the bread for bananas baked in spices and butter. Delicious!

6 bananas
1 teaspoon cinnamon
1 teaspoon nutmeg
1 tablespoon raisins or sultanas
2 tablespoons ghee or butter

Serve with
Whipped heavy cream (optional)

1 Preheat oven to 350°F.

2 Peel the bananas and slice into large chunks. Line the bananas in a baking dish. Sprinkle the spices and dried fruit on top.

3 Place chunks of butter or ghee over the bananas.

4 Bake for around 20 minutes or until the bananas are soft. Stir halfway through cooking to mix the spices and fruit with the oils from the fat.

PREPARATION TIME: 5 minutes
COOKING TIME: 20-30 minutes
SERVES: 4-5

Dark Chocolate Almond Cake

This is a rich, moist cake sweetened with honey. You'll only need a small slice to hit that chocolate craving.

3.5-ounce 70 to 85 percent dark
    chocolate bar
2 tablespoons raw honey
¾ cup butter
¾ cup ground almonds
3 eggs, separated
¼ teaspoon baking soda (optional)

PREPARATION TIME: 15 minutes
COOKING TIME: 50 minutes–1 hour
SERVES: 8-10

1 Preheat oven to 350°F.

2 Melt the chocolate, honey, and butter in a heat-proof glass bowl over a saucepan of simmering water to create a double boiler effect. Remove from the heat and stir in the almonds.

3 Beat the egg whites and yolks separately. Add the beaten egg yolks to the chocolate mixture and then slowly fold in the beaten egg whites. Alternatively, beat the eggs in a food processor until pale, then add to the melted ingredients and ground almonds.

4 Bake in an 8-inch cake pan for 50 minutes to 1 hour.

 TIP This cake has a very moist texture. To make a lighter cake, add ¼ teaspoon baking soda.

Chocolate Chestnut Fudge Cake

Using a chestnut puree in the cake mixture makes a fantastic fudgy cake that simply melts in your mouth. Your friends will think you've slaved for hours putting together this culinary masterpiece, but it actually takes about 15 minutes to prepare.

3.5-ounce 70 percent dark chocolate bar
6 eggs
8 ounces (1 stick) grass-fed butter
2 tablespoons raw honey or maple syrup
15-ounce can of chestnut puree

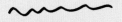

PREPARATION TIME: 15 minutes
COOKING TIME: 40-50 minutes
SERVES: 8-10

1 Preheat oven to 350°F.

2 Melt the chocolate, butter, and honey in a heat-proof glass bowl over a saucepan of simmering water to create a double boiler effect.

3 Remove from the heat and stir in the chestnut puree.

4 Whisk the eggs and fold into the mixture.

5 Pour into a 9½-inch springform pan and bake for 40 minutes.

6 After 30 minutes, start to check the cake by inserting a knife into the middle. It should not come out clean; rather, it should be sticky, as the middle of the cake is best moist.

7 When it's ready, remove the cake from the oven and serve warm.

8 Wrap the leftover cake in parchment paper and keep it in the fridge. Eaten cold, this cake is like a slab of rich chocolate fudge. Yum!

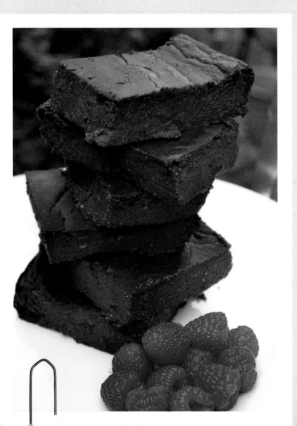

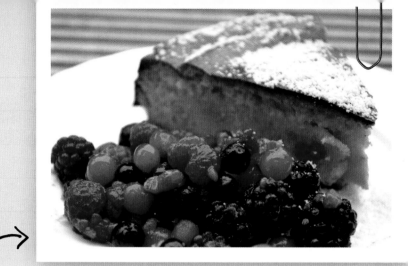

Portuguese Almond Cake

Here we replaced flour and sugar with some ground almonds and raw honey. This is a rather light cake—instead of the traditional almond syrup used in the Portuguese recipe, we like to serve it with some fresh seasonal berries.

6 eggs
2 tablespoons raw honey
1 cup ground almonds
1 teaspoon almond extract
1 teaspoon baking soda

Serve with
Fresh berries

1 Preheat oven to 350°F.

2 Beat the eggs on low with a hand or stand mixer. (A blender will also work.)

3 Add the ground almonds, honey, almond extract, and baking soda and continue to mix.

4 Bake in a 9½-inch round baking pan for 50 minutes to 1 hour. Check the cake after 45 minutes; the top of the cake should be golden brown and the middle slightly moist.

5 Once cooked, let the cake cool before serving.

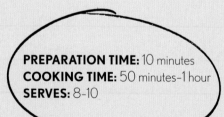

PREPARATION TIME: 10 minutes
COOKING TIME: 50 minutes–1 hour
SERVES: 8-10

Plum cake

A fruity and moist cake, perfect for afternoon tea.

4 eggs
6 ounces butter
¾ cup coconut sugar
  or 2 tablespoons raw honey
1 cup ground almonds
1 teaspoon vanilla extract
1 teaspoon baking soda
8-10 plums, pitted and sliced in half

PREPARATION TIME: 20 minutes
COOKING TIME: 50 minutes–1 hour
SERVES: 8-10

1 Preheat oven to 325°F.

2 Beat the eggs, butter, and coconut sugar or honey on low with a hand or stand mixer. (If you don't own a mixer, a blender will do.)

3 Add the ground almonds, vanilla extract, and baking powder and continue to mix.

4 Stir in the plum halves.

5 Bake in a 9½-inch round baking pan for 60 minutes. Check the cake by inserting a knife into the middle; it should come out clean.

6 Once cooked, let the cake cool slightly before serving.

MUM'S LEGENDARY ALMOND & PEAR TART

A fruity (and more palatable) take on Britain's traditional pork pie!

For the Pastry
1 cup ground almonds
3 ounces butter, softened

For the Filling
8 ounces (1 stick) butter
4 eggs
2 teaspoons almond extract
3 pears, cored and chopped
¾ cup coconut sugar
    (or 2 tablespoons raw honey)
1 cup ground almonds
1 teaspoon baking soda

Serve with
A spoonful of crème fraîche
(optional)

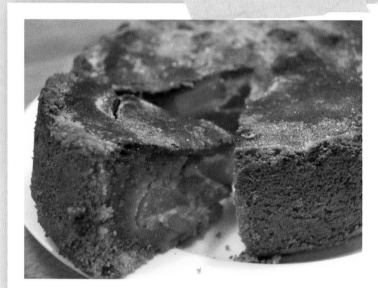

PREPARATION TIME: 10 minutes
COOKING TIME: 1 hour and 30 minutes
SERVES: 8-10

1 Preheat oven to 325°F.

2 Start by making the pastry. Place the ground almonds and butter in a bowl and use clean hands to mix together. (This can also be done in a food processor.) Squeeze the mixture together so it binds into a ball.

3 Place the pastry on a flat surface covered with parchment paper or a bread board dusted with ground almonds.

4 Flatten the pastry either using the palm of your hand or a rolling pin. The mixture will break up because it doesn't contain gluten, so it resembles more of a crumble. Do not worry, it will be fine once it is baked.

5 Now line an 8-inch springform pan with the crumbled pastry mixture. Treat it like Play-Doh and press it on the bottom and sides of the pan, around ¼ inch in thickness.

6 To make the filling, beat the remaining butter into the eggs, almond extract, and sugar (or honey) either by hand, using a hand whisk, or in a stand mixer until a light, fluffy mixture forms.

7 Add the ground almonds and 1 teaspoon baking soda, and mix again.

8 Place the chopped pears in the cake pan on top of the pastry lining. It should be filled roughly halfway with fruit.

9 Pour the almond cake mixture over the top.

10 Bake for 90 minutes. Check the cake after an hour; if the top of the cake is browning too quickly, cover it with foil.

11 Allow the cake to cool slightly; serve warm.

CHESTNUT COOKIES

Chestnut cookies are fantastic when you need a little crunch in your life. Chestnuts are a nutrient-rich source of starch, and the sweetness of the flour makes it great for baking. Here are six suggested cookie variations—feel free to come up with your own.

Basic Biscuit Recipe
4 ounces (½ stick) butter, softened
1 cup chestnut flour
1 egg

Variations
- ❄ **Ginger:** Add 2 teaspoons of ginger powder
- ❄ **Date and walnut:** Add 5 dates, finely chopped, and 2 ounces chopped walnuts
- ❄ **Apricot:** Add 8 unsulphured dried apricots, finely chopped
- ❄ **Cinnamon:** Add 1 teaspoon of cinnamon
- ❄ **Winter spice:** Add 1 teaspoon mixed spice and 2 tablespoons white raisins
- ❄ **Dark chocolate chip:** Add 2 ounces dark chocolate, finely chopped

1 Preheat oven to 350°F.

2 Rub the butter and chestnut flour together, either by hand or using a food processor.

3 Add your flavor of choice.

4 Add an egg to bind the biscuit mixture and mix again.

5 Place the dough on a flat surface dusted with some extra chestnut flour. Roll out the dough to a ¼-inch thickness using a rolling pin or a glass bottle.

6 Cut out biscuit shapes using a 2-inch cookie cutter or the rim of a drinking glass. Place biscuits onto a baking sheet lined with parchment paper or a little oil to prevent the biscuits from sticking.

7 Bake for 10-12 minutes or until golden brown around the edges.

8 Let the cookies cool before serving. Keep in an airtight container for up to 1 week.

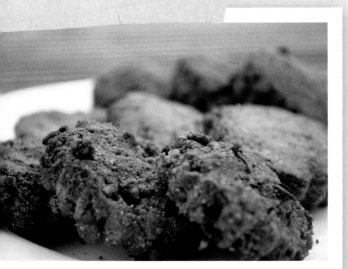

PREPARATION TIME: 10 minutes
COOKING TIME: 10-12 minutes
SERVES: 8-10

Chocolate-Dipped Strawberries

Not exactly the most technical recipe—just a simple, quick treat packed with antioxidants.

1 Break the dark chocolate into small pieces, and place in a heat-proof glass bowl set over a saucepan of simmering water to create a double boiler effect. Stir occasionally until the chocolate has melted (around 3-5 minutes). Remove the melted chocolate from the heat.

2 Line a baking sheet with parchment paper. One at a time, dip each strawberry into the dark chocolate, twirling to coat fully. Place the chocolate-dipped strawberries on the lined baking sheet.

3 Chill in the fridge for at least 15 minutes for the chocolate to set. Do not leave for much longer than 15 minutes, as condensation will start to form on the strawberries and moisten the chocolate. These are best served on the day they are made.

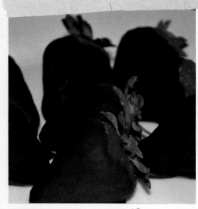

PREPARATION TIME: 10 minutes
COOKING TIME: 0 minutes
SERVES: 10

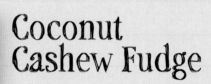

3.5-ounce 85 percent dark chocolate bar
7 ounces (or 1 carton) fresh strawberries

Coconut Cashew Fudge

This fudge is incredibly rich and makes the perfect accompaniment to an after-dinner espresso at parties. You can use different nut butters like macadamia, hazelnut, or almond.

1 Place all the ingredients in a bowl and mix well.

2 Line a small baking sheet or glass baking dish with parchment paper. Pour the mixture onto the paper and spread evenly until the mixture is about an inch thick.

3 Put into the refrigerator for 2-3 hours or until it becomes solid.

4 Cut into 1-inch squares and serve. Store in the refrigerator or freeze the remaining fudge.

8-ounce jar of cashew butter
6 tablespoons melted coconut oil
1-2 tablespoons honey
6 tablespoons cocoa powder
6 tablespoons unsulphured desiccated coconut

PREPARATION TIME: 10 minutes
CHILLING TIME: 2-3 hours
SERVES: 8-10

RESOURCES

SOURCING LOCAL INGREDIENTS

Sourcing locally means the ingredients that go into your meals are fresh and therefore have a higher nutrient content. Below we list a couple of reliable sites to help you find grass-fed foods, farmers markets, and health food stores in your area.

FARMERS MARKETS AND CO-OPS

✳ Local CSA Farmers Market Directory	LocalHarvest.org
✳ Organic Consumers Association	OrganicConsumers.org/foodcoops.htm

GRASS-FED FARMS

✳ Eat Wild	EatWild.com
✳ Tendergrass Farms	GrassFedBeef.org

HEALTH FOOD STORES

✳ Alfalfa's Market (Boulder, CO)	Alfalfas.com
✳ Bi-Rite Markets (San Francisco)	BiRiteMarket.com
✳ Sprouts (Southwest)	Sprouts.com
✳ The Fresh Market	TheFreshMarket.com
✳ Trader Joe's	TraderJoes.com
✳ Whole Foods	WholeFoodsMarket.com

SOURCING ONLINE

If there is nothing local or convenient for you, then consider buying direct from a farm online or from a meat delivery company. Here is a list of mostly US-based companies offering excellent Primal-approved products in various categories.

TRADITIONALLY CURED MEATS AND FISH

✳ Fork in the Road Foods	ForkInTheRoad.com
✳ Nick's Sticks	Nicks-Sticks.com
✳ Primal Pacs	PrimalPacs.com
✳ Slant Shack Jerky,	SlantShackJerky.com
✳ Steve's Paleo Goods	StevesPaleoGoods.com
✳ The New Primal	TheNewPrimal.com

MEAT, FISH, AND PRODUCE DELIVERY

✳ Brandon Natural Beef	BrandonNaturalBeef.com
✳ Diestel Turkey	DiestelTurkey.com
✳ North Star Bison	NorthStarBison.com
✳ Slanker's	TexasGrassfedBeef.com
✳ The Fruit Guys	FruitGuys.com
✳ Thompson River Ranch	ThompsonRiverRanch.com
✳ Topline Foods	TopLineFoods.com
✳ TX Organics	TxBarOrganics.com
✳ US Wellness Meats	GrasslandBeef.com
✳ Vital Choice	VitalChoice.com
✳ Wild Alaskan Salmon Company	Seabeef.com
✳ Wild Pacific Salmon	WildPacificSalmon.com

SPECIALTY ITEMS

These websites and stores are useful for good quality oils, nuts, spices, coconut products, and dairy:

✳ Artisana (coconut oils and nut butters)	ArtisanaFoods.com
✳ Bulk Foods (nuts and spices)	BulkFoods.com
✳ Green Pasture (oils)	GreenPasture.org
✳ iHerb (groceries, toiletries, supplements)	iHerb.com
✳ Lucero Olive Oil	LuceroOliveOil.com
✳ Living Nutz (nuts, fruits, seeds, spices)	LivingNutz.com
✳ Santa Barbara Chocolate	SantaBarbaraChocolate.com
✳ Nutiva (coconut, hemp, chia products)	Nutiva.com
✳ Pure Indian Foods (Indian groceries)	PureIndianFoods.com
✳ Tierra Farm (nuts, seeds, fruits, butters, fair trade coffee, and chocolate)	TierraFarm.com
✳ Tropical Traditions (coconut products)	TropicalTraditions.com
✳ You Bar (nutrition bars)	YouBars.com

LIFE-SAVING BOOKS & WEBSITES

The theories behind *The Paleo Primer* are corroborated by outstanding experts and nutritionists who have spent decades observing the scientific literature on nutrition and disease. They were the first to identify that the caveman diet provided an exceptional model for optimal health and disease prevention. As nutrition science evolves, so should you. Listed below are some leading authorities who work ceaselessly to establish the truth about human nutrition.

ROBB WOLF
A former research biochemist, Robb Wolf is the author of the *New York Times* bestseller *The Paleo Solution*. Buy this book! Wolf is the man behind the legendary podcast *The Paleo Solution* (episodes are available for free on iTunes). He will also go down in history for inventing the "caveman cocktail": the NorCal Margarita, made with 100 percent agave tequila, fresh lime, and soda water.
www.robbwolf.com

CHRIS KRESSER
Chris Kresser is a practitioner of integrative medicine and the man behind The Healthy Skeptic (now ChrisKresser.com). Kresser's articles detail all the current scientific debates surrounding nutrition and provide an informed, objective response. Life-changing purchases on his website include his Personal Paleo Code, Healthy Baby Code, and High Cholesterol Diet Plan wellness programs. Tune in to his free Revolution Health Radio podcast to get up to speed on the latest essential nutrition information.
www.chriskresser.com

MARK SISSON
A former endurance athlete and bestselling author of *The Primal Blueprint*, Mark Sisson is on a mission to empower people with the truth about health and wellness. Whenever you have a "Should I eat this?" moment, check out his website, Mark's Daily Apple. A walking encyclopedia of everything caveman, Sisson provides a fantastic lowdown on the pros and cons of almost any food you can think of. In addition to great recipes, blogs, and videos, there are some fantastic articles about how (and why) we should strive to live life like our ancestors did, enjoying hours of fun and playful movement while keeping stress and disease to a minimum.
www.marksdailyapple.com

PAUL AND SHOU-CHING JAMINET
Paul and Shou-Ching Jaminet are the husband-and-wife team who created the *Perfect Health Diet* after overcoming a number of health issues themselves. Paul is a former astrophysicist and Shou-Ching is a molecular biologist and cancer researcher. Their program is illustrated on page 38, and their website provides a fantastic insight into the use of nutritional supplements and "supplemental foods," including the recommendation for a daily dose of some antioxidant-rich dark chocolate. We aren't going to argue with that!
www.perfecthealthdiet.com

CHRIS MASTERJOHN

Chris Masterjohn is a former vegetarian who decided to pursue a doctorate in nutritional sciences, resulting in his becoming a true cholesterol expert. Before you start worrying about how many eggs you've had this week, get up to speed with the history, politics, and biochemistry of cholesterol. Follow his blog, The Daily Lipid, for an understanding of why cholesterol is vital to health. And once again, if you're still considering making an egg-white omelet, first check out his article, "The Incredible, Edible Egg Yolk."
www.cholesterol-and-health.com

CHARLES POLIQUIN

The Poliquin Performance website provides some fantastic blogs and articles by coach Charles Poliquin. Check out his lifestyle page for some highly effective nutrition philosophies and holistic health advice.
www.charlespoliquin.com

SÉBASTIEN NOËL

Sébastien Noël is a nutrition, fitness, and healthy lifestyle enthusiast who developed the popular website Paleo Diet Lifestyle. With articles covering popular topics such as nutrition and fertility, gut health, and immune function, Sébastien covers everything you could ever need to know about paleo foods, from the fat profile of every nut to some great recipes and cooking tips.
www.paleodietlifestyle.com

MIKE MAHLER

Mike Mahler is a strength trainer and hormone optimization researcher based in Las Vegas. His book, *Live Life Aggressively! What Self-Help Gurus Should Be Telling You,* provides great insight into hormone optimization via nutrition, exercise, and lifestyle. His website provides a fantastic online library of articles covering brain health, fat loss, and stress management.
www.mikemahler.com

KURT HARRIS

Kurt Harris is a practicing, board-certified radiologist and a senior member of the American Society of Neuroradiology, and has a lifelong interest in science and medicine and provides great commentary on his website. He developed a framework for healthy nutrition known as the Archevore Diet, a pastoral whole foods diet aiming to avoid the most hazardous foods that have developed from industrial processing.
www.archevore.com

SARAH MYHILL

Sarah Myhill is a private medical practitioner and Secretary of the British Society for Ecological Medicine. A keen advocate of the caveman diet, her fantastic website provides a wealth of information about maintaining and restoring good health. Dr. Myhill strongly encourages the practice of medicine which looks at the causes of health issues, focusing on nutrition, micronutrient status, allergies, and lifestyle changes. She provides access to extensive nutrition tests to help people take control of their health.
www.drmyhill.co.uk

METRIC CONVERSIONS

For our friends outside the United States, we offer the following metric conversion charts. These are not exact equivalents, but have been rounded up or down for easier measuring and work well with most recipes in this cookbook. However, when preparing baked goods, we strongly recommend that you visit one of the many food-related websites or smartphone app for a more precise conversion system specific to your country to ensure the best results. Regardless of the measuring system you use, the same system should be followed throughout.

U.S. MEASURES TO METRIC:
(Based on the approach to metric measures developed in the United States and Canada)

Ounces to grams: multiply ounces by 28.35
Pounds to grams: multiply pounds by 453.5
Cups to liters: multiply cups (or fraction thereof) by 0.24
Fahrenheit to Celsius: subtract 32 from Fahrenheit temperature, multiply by 5, then divide by 9

Liquid Measures (Volume) May be used to calculate spices in small quantities	
⅛ teaspoon	0.5 ml
¼ teaspoon	1 ml
½ teaspoon	2 ml
¾ teaspoon	4 ml
1 teaspoon	5 ml
1 tablespoon	15 ml
¼ cup	60 ml
⅓ cup	75 ml
½ cup	125 ml
⅔ cup	150 ml
¾ cup	175 ml
1 cup	250 ml
2 cups	500 ml
1 quart	1000 ml or 1 L
1 gallon	4 L

Weight Measures for solids, including meat, cheese, butter, flour, sugar	
½ ounce	15 g
1 ounce	25 g or 30 g
3 ounces	90 g
4 ounces	115 g or 125 g
8 ounces	225 g or 250 g
12 ounces	350 g or 375 g
16 ounces (1 pound)	450 g or 500 g
2¼ pounds	1 kg
5 pounds	2.5 kg

Oven Temperatures	
Fahrenheit	Celsius
300°	150°
325°	160°
350°	180°
375°	190°
400°	200°

NUTRITIONAL INFORMATION

Eating a paleo diet doesn't require that you count calories. However, we know some people like to track their daily intake of carbs and dietary fats. With that in mind, we offer the following nutritional values. But unlike processed foods that are pressed out by machines, home cooking is not entirely exact. For one, produce comes out of the garden in various sizes. And it may be that you desire a larger fish fillet or steak, a larger serving of greens, or you determine to be less liberal with the sweetener. To that end, the following nutritional values are estimates, gathered from the online food tracking source FitDay.com.

All the recipes are calculated at single portions. In recipes that state a range, say, 1 to 2 teaspoons of a specific herb or serves 4 to 5 people, we elected to calculate the less caloric option, so 1 teaspoon or 5 servings would be calculated for these examples. Recipes that call for "a handful" of greens have been calculated at 1/2 cup. Fish fillets are calculated at 5 ounces and steaks are calculated at 6 ounces. Dips, oils, and condiments are calculated at single servings of 2 tablespoons.

	CALORIES	FAT (G)	CARBS (G)	PROTEIN (G)
Avocado Breakfast Bowl	596	34	11	64
BLT	287	10	2	26
Baked Squash Discs	91	0	24	2
Baked Tomato Salmon	285	10	15	36
Bangers and Mash	518	34	27	25
(without cabbage)	327	23	26	6
(with buttered Savoy cabbage)	397	27	33	9
Beef and Creamy Cauliflower	202	4	2	33
Beef and Mustard Burgers	270	18	0	25
Blackberry Apple Crumble (without cream)	444	35	30	10
Breadless Butter Pudding	187	5	37	2
Breakfast Burger	275	20	12	14
Breakfast Calzone	429	33	7	54
Breakfast Stir-Fry	415	13	7	15
Bubble and Squeak (1 cup)				
(sweet potato)	137	10	20	2
(broccoli)	35	2	3	1
(carrots)	42	2	5	0
(zucchini)	20	2	0	0
(celery)	30	2	2	0
Buttered Savoy Cabbage				
(without bacon)	56	3	7	2
(with bacon)	70	4	7	3
Butternut Smash	51	1	13	1
Caribbean Jerk Salmon	264	13	2	33
Cauliflower Mash	83	5	9	3
Cauliflower Pizza	345	23	13	23

	CALORIES	FAT (G)	CARBS (G)	PROTEIN (G)
Cauliflower Rice	97	5	12	5
Celeriac Chips	109	7	11	2
Chestnut Cookies (without additions)	124	10	9	1
Chestnut Tea Cake	94	9	7	1
Chicken Vindaloo	551	27	18	53
Chili Con Cauliflower	609	38	16	51
Chili Roasted Macadamias	221	53	4	2
Chocolate Chestnut Fudge Cake	447	32	38	4
Chocolate-Dipped Strawberries (each)	59	3	7	0
Chocolate Macadamias	252	21	17	3
Chunky Zucchini Chips	29	3	2	1
Cinnamon Coconut Squash	179	11	23	3
Citrus Ceviche with Tomato and Avocado (without onion)	367	22	8	32
(with onion)	405	22	20	34
(with jalapeño)	422	22	42	67
Citrus Fries	37	0	8	1
Coconut Cashew Fudge	250	23	11	5
Coconut Comfort Curry	469	41	10	20
Creamy Green Omelet	466	39	11	21
(with ½ cup chicken)	626	48	11	39
(with ½ cup fish)	592	40	11	47
Crispy Stuffing Balls	267	16	10	20
Crunchy Nut Coconut Flakes	533	25	19	7
Dark Chocolate Almond Cake	423	32	33	5
Egg-Stuffed Toms	457	39	14	15
Everyday Chicken Curry	509	19	24	62
Fish, Chips, and Mushy Peas	573	30	37	40
Fish Fingers	277	15	2	34
Fish in a Blanket	314	14	3	20
Grass-Fed Steak with Garlic Fries and Béarnaise Sauce				
(without Béarnaise sauce)	442	20	25	42
(with Béarnaise sauce)	709	48	27	46
Guacamole (2 tablespoons)				
(without onion)	128	10	10	3
(with onion)	137	10	12	3
Homemade Kettle Chips	77	3	13	1
Homemade Mayonnaise	249	28	0	0
Italian Meatballs	492	26	32	38
Kale and Chorizo Mash	473	32	29	17
Ketchup (2 tablespoon)	24	0	3	0

	CALORIES	FAT (G)	CARBS (G)	PROTEIN (G)
Lamb and Cumin Burgers	276	19	2	24
Lebanese-Style Beef				
(without cauliflower)	669	41	14	60
(with cauliflower)	705	44	16	61
Lemon and Olive Chicken Tagine	452	2	14	2
Lemon and Thyme Baked Carrots	38	0	9	1
Lightning Lamb Kebab (each)	240	11	8	26
Liver and Bacon	517	23	19	56
Liver Dippy Egg	514	20	10	70
LiverPâte	263	20	3	19
Mackerel and Sweet Potato Fish Cakes	456	27	27	29
Man Maker Pie	514	20	10	70
(with beef)	639	38	29	46
(with lamb)	656	45	29	35
Matt's Big Beefy Onion and Chorizo	350	24	3	29
Matt's Mighty Scotch Eggs	260	20	4	16
Mediterranean Bake	216	15	17	7
(without goat cheese)	176	10	21	3
(with goat cheese)	236	15	27	7
Moules Marinara	422	10	10	37
Movie Mix	480	23	34	5
Mum's Legendary Almond & Pear Tart (without cream)	457	40	22	7
Mustard Seed Salmon	492	35	10	38
"OMG! Where's the Protein?" Salad	455	40	16	16
Oil Infusions (2 tablespoons olive oil)	239	27	0	0
Omega Breakfast Bake	346	25	3	29
Pan-Fried Spicy Mackerel	348	23	1	33
Parsley Salmon and Poached Eggs	340	15	3	46
Pesto Pork Cupcakes				
(without topping)	157	11	0	13
(with topping)	160	12	0	13
Plum Cake	268	22	17	4
Poach an Egg, How to (1 egg)	74	5	0	6
Pockets of Power	158	9	10	10
Portuguese Almond Cake	126	8	11	4
Preserved Lemons (per lemon)	24	0	8	0
Primal Shepherd's Pie	317	19	16	22
Quick and Easy Tomato Sauce (2 tablespoons)	29	2	4	0
Quick-Cook Chive Scrambled Eggs and Bacon	381	30	4	25
Quick Piri Piri Chicken	617	12	3	16

	CALORIES	FAT (G)	CARBS (G)	PROTEIN (G)
Shrimp Cocktail	283	17	5	28
Soaked Sun-Dried Tomatoes, oil drained (1 piece)	15	1	1	0
Spicy Carrot Chips	107	7	11	1
Spinach, Sun-dried Tomatoes, and Pine Nuts	45	3	3	2
Sun-Dried Stuffed Chicken Breast	366	24	3	35
Sweet and Spicy Chicken	272	13	5	32
Sweet Garlic Shrimp	314	25	8	16
Sweet Potato Wedges	308	16	39	5
Tarragon Turkey Burgers	254	13	7	27
Tarragon Roast Chicken and Chestnut Stuffing				
(without stuffing)	594	9	4	16
(with stuffing)	1097	34	40	48
Thai Burgers				
(with turkey)	233	13	2	26
(with chicken)	237	13	2	26
(with pork)	291	20	2	25
Thai Chicken and Spring Onion Rice	427	24	24	34
Thai Mussels	530	32	11	24
Thai Sea Bass Supper	234	8	6	33
Toasted Coconut	36	3	2	0
Toasted Walnuts (1 ounce)	98	10	2	2
Tuna Avo Egg	528	25	9	69
Turkey, Chestnut, Rosemary Burgers	186	9	10	17
Turkey Coconut Curry	959	58	40	77
Turkey Toast	285	17	0	31
Turmeric and Black Pepper Chicken with Rainbow Veg	463	28	26	30
Vegetable Kebabs	125	3	25	2
Vegetable Spaghetti				
(medium Zucchini, large carrot, ½ cup squash)	66	2	11	2
Zucchini and Chive Fritters	319	9	6	11
Toasted Coconut	36	3	2	0
Toasted Walnuts (1 ounce)	96	9	2	2
Tuna Avo Egg	528	25	9	69
Turkey, Chestnut, Rosemary Burgers	186	9	10	17
Turkey Coconut Curry	959	58	40	77
Turkey Toast	285	17	0	31
Turmeric and Black Pepper Chicken with Rainbow Veg	463	28	26	30
Vegetable Kebabs	125	3	25	2
Vegetable Spaghetti				
(medium zucchini, large carrot, ½ cup squash)	66	2	11	2
Zucchini and Chive Fritters	319	9	6	11

RECIPE INDEX

SUBJECT INDEX

macadamias, 54
macronutrients, 21-23
Marine Stewardship Council (MSC), 51
Masterjohn, Chris, 50
meals, 45
metabolism, 12-13, 19, 21, 23, 28, 30, 43
micronutrients, 21-23, 31, 32
mindful eating, 1-19
minerals, 8, 21-23,27, 29, 31, 35,37-38, 42, 50, 54-55
   calcium, 23, 27, 42, 50
   magnesium, 22, 23, 31-32, 42, 54
   potassium, 22, 31-32, 42
   selenium, 32, 54
   sodium, 31, 58
   zinc, 22-23, 27, 31-32, 50, 54
My Plate, 23

N
Noël, Sebastien, 56
nuts, 52-54, 60-61

O
Omega-3, 30, 50-51, 53, 61
Omega-6, 9, 30, 39, 50, 53-54, 61
organic, 42, 47, 50, 52-53, 55,57-58
   Clean Fifteen, 57
   Dirty Dozen, 57

P
paleo diet, 7-9, 22, 61
peanuts, 39
phytates, 23, 27, 30, 36, 38-39
polycystic ovarian syndrome (PCOS), 4, 13
polyunsaturated vegetable oil. *See also omega-6, omega-3, and fats and oils*. 15, 22, 26, 29, 52-53
preservatives, 12, 15, 28, 30
Primal lifestyle. *See paleo diet.*
proteins, 27, 29, 50

S
salt. *See also sodium*. 15, 58
seafood. *See also fish.* 51, 60
shopping, 18, 55, 57, 59, 60,
Sisson, Mark, 3, 27, 45
skin issues, 14, 21
sleep requirements, 12-13, 41. 43
sodium. *See also salt*. 31, 58
soy beans. *See also legumes*. 39

spices. See also herbs. 5, 7, 15, 58, 61
stabilizers, 28
starches, 28
   safe starches, 38
sugar. *See also sweeteners*. 9, 12 ,15, 21-22, 25-26, 28-30, 35
sugar free. *See also artificial sweetener*. 28, 46, 56, 61
sulfites, 28
Sutter, Hannah, 24-25
sweeteners. *See also sugar*. 15, 28, 30, 35, 56, 61

T
tea, 42, 47
toxins, 14-15, 30, 43
trans fats. *See also fats and oils*. 15, 29-30

V
vegetables, 7, 21, 23, 31, 37, 39, 45-46, 55-56
vitamins, 21-22, 29, 31-32, 50, 55
   B vitamins, 27, 39, 32
   vitamin A, 22, 23, 27, 29, 31, 32
   vitamin C, 27, 31, 32
   vitamin D, 22, 27, 29, 31, 32
   vitamin E, 22, 29, 31, 32
   vitamin K, 22, 29, 31, 32

W
Whittingstall, Hugh Fearnley, 51
whole grains. *See grains.*
withdrawals. *See cravings.*
Wolf, Robb, 18, 27

Y
yogurt, 32, 39, 53

Z
zucchini, 32

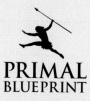

PRIMAL
BLUEPRINT

Other books by Primal Blueprint Publishing

MARK SISSON

The Primal Blueprint: *Reprogram your genes for effortless weight loss, vibrant health, and boundless energy*

The Primal Blueprint 21-Day Total Body Transformation: *A step-by-step gene reprogramming action plan*

The Primal Blueprint 90-Day Journal: *A Personal Experiment (n=1)*

COOKBOOKS BY MARK SISSON AND JENNIFER MEIER

The Primal Blueprint Cookbook: *Primal, low carb, paleo, grain-free, dairy-free and gluten-free meals*

The Primal Blueprint Quick and Easy Meals: *Delicous, Primal-approved meals you can make in under 30 minutes*

The Primal Blueprint Healthy Sauces, Dressings, and Toppings: *Plus rubs, dips, marinades and other easy ways to transform basic natural foods into Primal masterpieces*

OTHER AUTHORS

Rich Food, Poor Food: *The Ultimate Grocery Purchasing System (GPS),* by Mira Calton, CN, and Jayson Calton, Ph.D.

ABOUT THE AUTHORS

Keris Marsden and Matt Whitmore are leading health and fitness professionals currently based in London. They are passionate about enhancing people's lives through the power of nutrition and exercise and have devoted their careers to training with leading experts in the health and fitness industry. After years of studying and exploring different theories on nutrition, they discovered an approach that quite simply made them feel fantastic. Using Primal/paleo principles, they have successfully guided their clients through the same life-changing experience, and ultimately decided to share their findings with as many people as possible, which is why this book was created.

While they share a love for exercise and nutrition (and each other!), there's one significant difference between them: Keris is a nutrition geek, and Matt loves cooking and being creative in the kitchen. Together they make the perfect team for putting together a nutrition and recipe book. One brings the knowledge and the other brings the taste.